'In the library of psychoanalytic studies, few address with such open candor as does this the *art* of clinical practice, the unforeseen challenges that confront every therapist. The abstinence principle exists to advance inquiry, not to serve as a cover story for the analyst's protection. In this master class, beginner and experienced analysts alike will discover challenges addressing what to hold back and what to reveal. Here, no rules are proclaimed, but the clarity of questions is richly sharpened. What could be better?'

Warren Poland, *author of* Intimacy and Separateness in Psychoanalysis

Self Disclosure and the Analytic Relationship

This book explores the inevitable intrusions of the analyst's personal life into clinical work and how to manage the challenges of self-disclosure, secrecy, and analytic identity within this context.

Are non-disclosure, abstinence, and neutrality realistic goals, or are they an artifact of an idealized analytic identification? Does self-disclosure of any sort by the analyst derail the analytic process and irrevocably damage the transference experience? Self-disclosure remains a compelling and central construct in the field of psychotherapy and psychoanalysis and there are few significant compendiums on this topic that explore the diversity of analytic voices. This book is an extraordinary collection of ideas from experienced psychoanalysts and psychotherapists who have wrestled with questions of self-disclosure from a theoretical, ethical, professional, and personal perspective. It describes the shifting landscape of the analytic field as it relates to self-disclosure, non-disclosure, the concept of neutrality and privacy, the limitations of the analytic frame, and the changing context of theoretical and global realities.

Self Disclosure and the Analytic Relationship will be a useful resource within all psychoanalytic contexts, including academic, clinical training, and post-graduate study.

Stephanie R. Brody, PsyD, is a supervising and training analyst at Boston Psychoanalytic Society and Institute and the author of *Entering Night Country: Psychoanalytic Reflections on Loss and Resilience* (2016).

Self Disclosure and the Analytic Relationship

Facing the Facts

Edited by Stephanie R. Brody

Routledge
Taylor & Francis Group
LONDON AND NEW YORK

Designed cover image: © Lisa Brody

First published 2027
by Routledge
4 Park Square, Milton Park, Abingdon, Oxon OX14 4RN

and by Routledge
605 Third Avenue, New York, NY 10158

Routledge is an imprint of the Taylor & Francis Group, an informa business

British Library Cataloguing-in-Publication Data
A catalogue record for this book is available from the British Library

ISBN: 978-1-032-95418-9 (hbk)
ISBN: 978-1-032-95103-4 (pbk)
ISBN: 978-1-003-58480-3 (ebk)

DOI: 10.4324/9781003584803

Typeset in Optima
by Apex CoVantage, LLC

To my family, friends, and colleagues – with endless gratitude for their generosity, understanding, and support

Contents

Acknowledgments

Dear Readers:

The idea for this book began in 2012, around the same time I initiated a discussion group on this topic at the national meetings of the American Psychoanalytic Association. In truth, the discussion group might have been on my mind for decades, but I wasn't quite ready. Though I had thought a lot about the topic and had experienced, more than once, the challenge of a self-disclosure dilemma, my personal fortitude did not yet permit me the freedom to tackle my colleagues, let alone a group.

But the facts kept streaming into my awareness: another pregnant therapist, another declining analyst, another provocative question, another internet search. My own medical event forced me to understand that I was more hesitant to open up to my colleagues than I was to my patients. And the literature that addressed the theoretical background for clinical decision-making seemed rigid and old-fashioned. There are very few professional forums where clinicians can safely discuss the numerous and tricky moments that are inevitable. Was it possible to wrestle with the choices, respond to the unthinkable, and contend with the unavoidable? What follows was the first effort to summarize the goal of the discussion group:

> *Currently, there are few educational forums for clinicians to receive training in the specific impact of personal self-disclosure within the context of the clinical relationship. While theoretical ideas regarding the significance of neutrality have long held meaning, the limitations of neutrality are significant when a fact about the clinician cannot be hidden – situations where the analyst's personal vulnerability may interfere with consistency or lead to patient curiosity. The inevitability of such an event requires preparation for clinical impacts and the professional and ethical responsibilities that are inherent during the close process work of psychoanalysis and psychotherapy. Anticipating these life events, and planning potential responses, is essential to remain effective throughout our professional careers.*

While this description effectively fulfilled the criteria for a professional meeting, the reality of our discussions was more nuanced, risky, and forceful. Each meeting had an honesty to it – a sense of power that comes with the experience of hearing a first-person account, a story that comes directly from the reporter. Though many more examples of personal disclosure could be in this collection, there were limits. Indeed, not everyone who has contributed to this book had an opportunity to present to the discussion group, and not everyone who presented to the group is included in the compilation. In every case, the reader is invited to explore a deeply challenging, meaningful, and often professionally altering experience.

The personal narratives reflect the complexity of the self-disclosure conundrum. The vantage point is flexible, pivoting from clinician to patient, from time past, to time present. The clinicians who have contributed their stories have struggled with maintaining, balancing, protecting, and opening their personal boundaries. They have also been on the receiving end of other clinicians who refused to share, or clients who refused to be barred entry. In each case, there is no right or wrong approach – only the genuine effort by every clinician to keep their client, or themselves useful and aware during a time of clinical meaning. As I was collecting the submissions, I tried to create thematic sections, loosely using words like concealment, transparency, flexibility, penetration, and accommodation – rearranging topics and authors to find their closest points of overlap. But it was hard to make final decisions – each chapter seemed to fit into more than one category, and no one word accurately described the theme for each author. Like a deck of cards, the whole set might have been shuffled in such a way that a new motif would emerge out of stories that reflected separate times, or theoretical ideas. Ultimately, it is fair to say that though each story is unique, the dilemma of disclosure is the theme that relates all of them.

Here are the sections:

1 Facing (or not facing) the Facts
2 What Cannot Be Hidden
3 Transparency and Porous Boundaries
4 Hidden, Found, Evolved

As you explore the personal narratives that follow, please note and admire the deep transparency of each contributor. Their original agreement to present to a discussion group[1] was a commitment to openness and risk. Not only did they agree to field penetrating questions from strangers, colleagues, and friends, but they also showed faith in my promise to them that controversial moments, strong opinions, and theoretical divides would occur in a safe surround, and there would be no personal attacks (there never was one). The discussion group did not seek to establish right or wrong, but rather to address how surprise and uncertainty can affect our work. The mission was to expand our understanding of the subtleties of human relationships in these difficult moments, to observe the nuances of action and empathy, and to reflect on the power of the relationship itself. We committed to maintaining dialogue, even when there was confusion, difference of opinion, or uncertainty. We acknowledged that we can never know how moments of vulnerability will unfold.

The pages that follow represent an original reflection with an additional disclosure – what has changed since the memorable event, and perhaps, what has not. I am pleased that the distinguished colleagues who agreed to present at the discussion group can be included in the permanent archive that will be this book. Each author has obtained permission from and/or has sufficiently disguised any client that has been represented in their contribution. Perhaps more tellingly, this collection is itself a series of self-disclosures by each author with the shared hope that their experiences may illuminate and penetrate the ongoing enigma of self-disclosure.

I hope their wisdom will be received with gratitude by those who take the time to read these pages. Personally, I am grateful for their enthusiasm and responsiveness – the invitation to participate in a book project was unexpected, and for many, the original presentations had been shelved. The authors have proved to be wonderful and generous collaborators, willing to revisit past events, with additional meaning based on clinical practice, and the passage of time. They offer differing perspectives. Indeed, it is my hope that this book will invite you to wonder what you would have done, and how it would have felt, had you found yourself in the same situation that unfolded in these stories. With some certainty, I can say, pay attention, because it is more than likely that one day, you will find yourself there.

Contributors

Anne Adelman, PhD, is a clinical psychologist, supervising and training analyst, and Institute Dean at the Washington Baltimore Center for Psychoanalysis, and a Teaching Analyst at the Contemporary Freudian Society. Dr. Adelman is the Editor of *JAPA Review of Books*, where she launched two feature columns called "Why I Write" and "What I'm Reading Now", Dr. Adelman is co-chair of the New Directions in Writing Program and is coauthor and editor of four books, including, published in 2022, *When The Garden Isn't Eden: More Psychoanalytic Stories from Life*, with Kerry Malawista and Linda Kanefield (Columbia University Press, 2022), along with several published papers and chapters. Dr. Adelman maintains a private practice in Chevy Chase, MD.

Michele Baker, MD, is a psychoanalyst and lecturer at Harvard University School of Medicine. She teaches at the Boston Psychoanalytic Society and Institute and supervises at Beth Israel Deaconess Medical Center in Boston. She has a private practice in Brookline, MA.

Stephanie R. Brody, Psy.D., is a training and supervising analyst at Boston Psychoanalytic Society and Institute, and Clinical Associate/Attending Psychologist at McLean Hospital in Belmont, MA, and Instructor in Psychology in the Department of Psychiatry, Harvard Medical School. She is the author of *Entering Night Country: Psychoanalytic Reflections on Loss and Resilience* (2016) and co-editor (with Fran Arnold) of *Psychoanalytic Perspectives on Women and their Experience of Desire, Ambition and Leadership* (2019). She maintains a private practice in Lexington, MA.

Robin A. Deutsch, PhD, is a training and supervising analyst and faculty at the San Francisco Center for Psychoanalysis. She is the Editor of *Traumatic Ruptures: Abandonment and Betrayal in the Analytic Relationship*, Routledge, 2014. She has presented on the subject of analytic identity, therapist subjectivity, and analyst aging and death. She has a private practice of psychoanalysis, psychotherapy, and consultation in Oakland, CA.

Linda Emanuel, MD, PhD, is a training analyst and on the faculty of the Chicago Psychoanalytic Institute, and is a member of the Boston Psychoanalytic Society and Institute. Professor Emerita of Northwestern, she was formerly the Center Director at Northwestern's Feinberg School of Medicine, where she focused on end-of-life care. She is currently engaged in research on existential maturation.

Cary Friedman, MD, is a training and supervising analyst and President-Elect at the Boston Psychoanalytic Society and Institute. He has written and spoken extensively about GLBTQ+ topics in psychoanalysis. He maintains a private practice in Cambridge, MA.

Holly Friedman Housman, LICSW, is currently a faculty member at the Boston Psychoanalytic Society and Institute, where she is also Chair of the Board of Trustees. She is a member and has been an active participant in the American Psychoanalytic Association Program Committee. She was an instructor, part-time, in the Department of Psychiatry, Harvard Medical School from 1982 to 2024. She has a private practice in Cambridge, MA.

Jane V. Kite, PhD, is currently a training and supervising analyst at the Boston Psychoanalytic Society and Institute and a member of the San Francisco Center for Psychoanalysis. She is an active participant in the American Psychoanalytic Association (Program Committee) and the International Psychoanalytic Association (North American Co-Chair, 2019 meeting on Femininity, currently a member of the Ethics committee), and an Associate Editor of *JAPA*. She has an abiding interest in the concept of character in psychoanalysis, and more recently what we actually mean by "ethics" in psychoanalytic discourse. She has a private practice in Cambridge, MA.

Susan Pasternak, DMH, is a psychoanalyst affiliated with The Boston Psychoanalytic Society and Institute. She currently has a private practice in New York City, where she works with individuals, couples, and families. Additionally, she volunteers at The Exodus Transition Community in Harlem, New York, treating previously incarcerated individuals.

Joseph Schwartz, PhD, is a licensed psychologist and psychoanalyst in private practice in Cambridge, MA. He is past Chair of the Board of Trustees of the Boston Psychoanalytic Society and Institute, Inc., where he is also on the faculty. Dr. Schwartz has a private practice in Cambridge, MA.

Karen E. Starr is a clinical psychologist and psychoanalyst. She is on the faculty at the New York University Postdoctoral Program in Psychotherapy and Psychoanalysis. In addition to numerous journal articles and book chapters, Dr. Starr is the author of *Repair of the Soul: Metaphors of Transformation in Jewish Mysticism and Psychoanalysis* (2008); co-author with Lewis Aron of *A Psychotherapy for the People: Toward a Progressive Psychoanalysis* (2013); and co-editor with Jill Bresler of *Relational Psychoanalysis and*

Psychotherapy Integration (2015). Dr. Starr maintains a private practice in New York City and Great Neck, New York.

Pratyusha Tummala-Narra, PhD, is a professor of counseling, developmental, and educational psychology at Boston College. Her research and scholarship focus on the psychology of immigration and trauma and culturally informed psychoanalytic psychotherapy. She is also a clinical psychologist in independent practice. Dr. Tummala-Narra is a Consulting Editor for *Psychoanalytic Dialogues* and for the *American Psychologist*. She has served as a member of the American Psychoanalytic Association Holmes Commission on Racial Equality, and in several leadership roles in the American Psychological Association (APA), including the APA Presidential Task Force on Immigration, the APA Task Force on Re-envisioning the Multicultural Guidelines, and the APA Presidential Task Force on Trauma and Grief. She is the author of *Psychoanalytic Theory and Cultural Competence in Psychotherapy* (2016), the editor of *Trauma and Racial Minority Immigrants: Turmoil, Uncertainty, and Resistance* (2021), and co-author of *Applying Multiculturalism: An Ecological Approach to the Multicultural Guidelines* (2023), all published by the American Psychological Association. Dr. Tummala-Narra is the recipient of numerous awards and honors, including being listed among the top 2% of Highly Cited Scholars Worldwide (Stanford University Report).

Note

1 All of the authors, except for Dr. Tummala-Narra, originally presented a version of their contribution during the meetings of the American Psychoanalytic Association in a discussion group that I organized called Facing the Facts: Self Disclosure and the Analytic Relationship.

Introduction

Self Disclosure and the Analytic Relationship: Facing the Facts

Stephanie R. Brody

Introduction

To locate and identify the paradox of our profession, one need look no further than the topic of self-disclosure. Psychoanalysis, indeed, every form of psychotherapy, relies on the patient's willingness to reveal, to share the intimate details of one's life, and the feelings that have brought them to therapy. But it is fair to say that even the most motivated patient may be detoured by inhibitions – a stockpile of obstructions that interfere with such an endeavor. Psychoanalysis is especially attuned to the idea that full disclosure, a conscious narrative of deep personal experience, is likely impossible. Whether it is due to shame or fear of judgment, much can remain hidden. Secrecy can act as conscious self-protection or be set in motion by a more unconscious defensive strategy. Any person engaged in the psychotherapy process will ultimately discover how much is being held back or has been concealed.

One of the great strengths and unique premises of psychoanalysis is that conscious and unconscious mental activity, what makes us think and feel, the core of our identity, can be uncovered, even if hidden. Our technique centers on the use of fantasy, dreams, free association, transference/countertransference, and repetitive patterns of interpersonal relationships. We rely on the use of metaphor, the signals that escape words, and the structures that bend in the face of desire and unmet needs. Coaxed into the dyadic space, disclosures become meaningful and potent facilitators of change. That our patients sign on and commit to the process is not because they agree to the uncovering or even because they understand how it will happen. They are seeking help with emotional pain. But as the therapeutic relationship evolves, the value of this profound and intimate process of disclosure, how the resistance or defiance moves into comprehension, cooperation and commitment, is a hallmark of progress and a relevant mutative factor within the process.

But alongside this complicated and ongoing commitment, an odd lopsidedness becomes evident and leads us to another psychoanalytic truth. The psychoanalyst is meant to be obscure to the patient. The ideas of anonymity and neutrality have long held that there is a therapeutic "value" in mystery. The psychoanalyst, in their search for the psychic reality of the patient, is

DOI: 10.4324/9781003584803-1

dedicated to a therapeutic life of opacity, to be a blank canvas upon which the patient will draw their perceptions, feelings, and beliefs about their analyst – without the imposition of facts. Within most psychoanalytic settings, questions and curiosity about the analyst's personal life are expected. Considered a tool of the trade, these inquires offer a path to additional understanding of the patient's inner life. Some questions are answered, some deflected, but the psychoanalytic aim is always to understand the patient's curiosity, and to collaborate on meaning making, whether or not a concrete answer is forthcoming. In the traditional version of analytic theory, in the historical ideal,[1] the analyst, seeking full disclosure from the patient, works to maintain a vault-like impenetrability of anonymity around herself. Unlike almost every other interpersonal relationship, in psychoanalysis, the expectation of openness is conceived as one-sided, and analytic disclosures have historically been regarded as unfortunate leaks in a system, much like a prolapsed cardiac valve that requires repair. However, over the past decades, while psychoanalytic anonymity remains part of the conversation, it is also regarded as a flawed, if impossible, ideal. The communication of personal meaning, from the comportment of the analyst herself, to the office furnishings, to the digitized content of one's online life, are recognized as open territory. Though not always comfortable, their presence in the analytic space cannot be avoided. Non-verbal signals, questions and silence, often convey conscious and unconscious interest, approval, or criticism. Patients scrutinize changes, listen to our breathing, notice a raised eyebrow, a laugh, or a fatigued sigh.

Inevitably, over a lifetime of shared history, even more information will emerge. After many decades of psychoanalytic dictum, there is an acknowledgment that even the most conscientious practitioner cannot lock all the gates. Our understanding of this impossibility comes from our own craft – the art of finding meaning and locating communications that arise from what operates outside of conscious awareness. We acknowledge that what is intentional and unintentional cannot always be known, at first. And the construction of our process requires the acceptance of this, even for the analyst – and especially in the context of the dyad. Many of us agree that it is more likely that a fact will surface than not – but none of us agree on exactly what to do when it happens.

The irony is inescapable. Though we wish to conceal, even agreeing that secrecy can harden clarity in the transference, the challenge to our privacy should be regarded as inevitable. Our patients will seek to know us, and over many hours, they *will* know us: the personal factors that contribute to their experience, the subtle qualities that set us apart or connect us, attributes of our personality, will be part of the relationship. Some may like what they discover, others may deny what they see. Some will outright reject the premise of our mystery, especially because the one-sidedness feels unfair. Assuming that there are qualities that we share does not mean that we are the same, especially when a patient's battles resonate with our own. But in every instance, how the dyad addresses an observation, a fantasy, or a fact becomes a valuable feature of the work. The analyst's openness to the possibility that curiosity can oscillate in the dyad, a confidence that all disclosures, some invited, intentional, or forced, will occur, or a sudden awareness of an unbidden disclosure – will provide moments of opportunity that can and should lead to exploration in the dyad. Though challenging to the unprepared analytic dyad, their presence can define, disrupt, or deepen a treatment. Mutual exploration is often an unexpected benefit of the process. But opinions differ.

In my book *Entering Night Country* (Brody, 2016), I have described some of the perspectives that have caused such strife, uncertainty, and tension in our field. Without considering the irony that analytic work is meant to root out what is hidden in our patients, while simultaneously avoiding access to what is hidden by the analyst, therapist non-disclosure, otherwise labeled *anonymity*, has evolved over the decades. The classical perspective argued that any self-disclosure risks the purity of the transference, and the patient's primary position in the treatment would be damaged by any disclosure. In an effort to preserve anonymity and neutrality, and to allow for the complexity of unconscious process, fantasy, and transference to unfold, the analyst was advised to always avoid any disclosure.

Ideas about therapist self-disclosure have been evolving for many decades out of necessity, opportunity and demand. The change reflects an acknowledgment that the analytic frame is permeable, and that psychoanalytic technique, the clinical praxis, cannot conform to such sterility. The version of the analyst as a "blank slate" is regarded as off putting, an analytic caricature, despite its meaningful intention. Our patients do not understand the theoretical objectives, or why personal information about the analyst is taboo. Why are certain questions allowed and others not: education, technique, experience? How about marital status, religion, ethnicity, or sexual orientation? Many clinicians have developed personal policies about what they share, what is comfortable, what patients have the right to know, and what is private. When the analyst divulges a useful interpretation, shares concerns about the patient, or reacts to a patient, it becomes more complicated. What is too much or too little information? When will the line be drawn? Though we focus on the patient as a therapeutic priority, we still seem to struggle with what to do when information collection shifts from the patient to the analyst/therapist.

It is useful to look at the self-disclosure as:

> an inevitable aspect of the dyad where disclosures of all kinds occur on many different levels of awareness, conscious and unconscious. The co-created space, even one that is skewed towards the therapist, would be regarded as a legitimate opportunity for an exploration of the interior world of the patient as well as the meaning of relational patterns. An argument might be made that non-disclosure in certain circumstances challenges the integrity of the therapeutic relationship.

> Without including the patient as part of the collaboration or negotiation, such decisions (to maintain secrecy) might be regarded as privileging the dominating authority of the analyst to decide what is or isn't relevant to the patient.
>
> (Brody, 2016, p. 136)

In relational/interpersonal theory, analytic self-disclosure may be referred to as "expressive participation", a term favored by Donnel Stern (Stern, 2020, p. 541). He notes that "the question (of) whether the analyst's experience is revealed to the patient is decided by the analyst's estimation of the relational context of the moment. There ceases to be a good reason to enforce analytic anonymity as policy– although the desirability of analytic restraint, of course, remains" (Stern, 2020, p. 541). And yet, there remains ongoing and interesting differences in the application of new psychoanalytic theories and how the intrusion of an external event can affect the analytic dyad.

I have always thought that therapist self-disclosure exists along a continuum where either an overly rigid adherence to or thoughtless violation of therapeutic anonymity could be anti-therapeutic. For me, each dyad is a matrix of intersecting factors and co-created relational patterns that reflect the complexity of life. For the patient, the matrix encompasses factors such as history, diagnosis, transference themes, relational strengths, and vulnerabilities, as well as the stage of treatment. For therapists, the matrix encompasses the right to privacy, the impact of secrecy, the use of affective self-disclosure, and unavoidable factual self-disclosures. As these matrices intersect, evolve, and expand in intensity and meaning, it is clear that every dyad will be different and ever-changing.

Can the analytic frame ever avoid a breach?

I think it's fair to say that patients know things about us, even when they are not told explicitly. Sometimes, they don't even know that they know, or what they know, as communications do travel from one unconscious to another. In other situations, patients may perceive and not ask or ask and receive no answer; they may seek out information from other sources, or may respectfully wait until they are informed. Whatever evolves during the intimate relationship dyad, I feel with increasing confidence, that embedded transference patterns are unlikely to be disrupted by a fact or an unexpected event, though challenge remains. How does the dyad effectively care for and attend to a patient's needs and maintain therapeutic viability and competence in the face of inevitable incursions? Effective treatment, whatever the theoretical perspective, depends on a sensitivity to these possibilities. We know from experience that the praxis of our work rarely adheres exactly to the theory that may organize the treatment. We can acknowledge that our theoretical ideas are rarely applied consistently in our work, that the person of the analyst can affect the delivery of the method, the interactive process, and the capacity to address an uncomfortable moment. This includes how different clinicians will address self-disclosure when it occurs. Our task will be to acknowledge the challenge, and in an ongoing processing of the event, maintain, sustain, and deepen the dyadic connection and the therapeutic process, whatever has occurred.

Privacy and Disclosure

Now here, I submit a most personal and ironic truth. I am a very private person. The meaning of such a self-reflection cannot be lost on the readers of this book, analysts and therapists, searching for the wisdom of experience from others who have dealt with these moments of disclosure. This topic is personal for me. It has been on my mind when decades ago, as a pregnant clinician, the standard policy regarding disclosure was to hold back any announcement until my patients brought it up. That directive seemed to pose more impediments to good clinical treatment than sharing what could not be hidden: Each patient reacted differently to my announcement. Some were able to talk more freely than others about the powerful feelings of anger, abandonment, envy, and fear that emerged. Many expressed relief, awkwardly confessing uncertainty about what was appropriate to say, worried they would be humiliated if they thought I was pregnant, but had really "just gained weight". Murderous rage toward me and the baby showed up behind a thinly veiled "concern" for my well-being; expressions of joy and a chance to share good wishes heralded a unique role for a patient whose profound social isolation interfered with a chance to experience normal human contact. In the ensuing years, when other non-life-threatening events, some medical and some personal occurred, I addressed each differently, based on the event, on the level of disruption, on the patient, and on my own desire for privacy. Over the years, I have had a lot of practice.

But to be vague has no value here. The event that was *most* intrusive for me and my practice was the rare cancer of the parotid gland, a part of the body that usually fails to attract much attention. Though it was nonlethal, the surgery would change my appearance, certainly temporarily, possibly permanently. Frighteningly unpredictable. It was nothing short of miraculous that my doctor saved my facial nerve which, if severed, would have permanently paralyzed my capacity to smile or blink. I returned to work with the expectation that my treatment was complete. But then, a curve ball diagnosis necessitated radiation. The temporary asymmetry of my smile had not prepared me for the next phase – partial hair loss, a sunburned face, and a chronically dry mouth. The radiation erased my taste buds for several weeks – food was dry as straw and tasted that way. I lost weight.

The position I took with my patients, to disclose the facts, did not represent a specific theoretical or technical school of thought. I consulted with supervisors, my analyst, and I did what made sense to me, what resonated with my analytic style. I needed to tell the truth, as best as I could, even though I knew it would be hard. The intersection between the actual facts and the dynamic uncertainty created a space that now seems uniquely analytic. Precisely attuned to the experience and dilemmas of life, I sought to create safety in the unknown and to maintain a connection within uncertainty; to make the most of the power we have while respecting our limitations and our helplessness. I needed to accept that I could be human (fallible) and also analytic (helpful) – a pivotal dimension of my new therapeutic identity.[2]

My situation, and how I chose to deal with it, elicited strong responses from colleagues. A paper[3] that resulted from my experience was rejected by a number of journals. Reviewers seemed split on its merit, alternately expressing outrage and praise, each side arguing their certainty. Our analytic community has strong opinions about what is right and what isn't. The intimacy of psychoanalysis, the possibility of exposure, uniquely places the clinician in the intersection of personal privacy, intimacy, transparency, and I would add, integrity. How will we navigate this unusual combination of factors that can upend a sense of stability and comfort?

Why have we wrestled so arduously with this impossible wish to remain obscure to those who are so close? I have suggested that anonymity as an argument for non-disclosure serves another purpose: It conveys the false belief that the analyst may be protected "from the enactment of his or her own internal process . . . and provides an essential fortifying barricade against the forces of the unconscious (that) exert influence on the analyst's conscious treatment behavior" (Brody, 2016, p. 135). This can only be aspirational.

More significant, and perhaps more difficult for the analyst to absorb, is another fact – both dreaded and inevitable: Analysts are human and thus vulnerable to human frailties. I have wondered if non-disclosure has been used to perpetuate a "collusion in illusion" (Brody, 2016, p. 105) – a form of professional denial that preserves a belief in our invulnerability and denies our patients a meaningful clinical opportunity. When one of these moments of analytic disclosure, subtle or dramatic, becomes part of the process, the patient's history is animated by contact with the analyst. The powerful meaning that becomes accessible can uncover a previously unknown emotional landscape. When actual or imagined attacks on the analyst's physical or emotional wellbeing enter the dyadic space, an overreliance on reassurance, or assertions of immunity, do not serve the exploratory value of analysis. The analyst's denials or minimization of our patient's observations, associations, or conscious and unconscious symbolic communications only serve to sustain the hapless illusion that the analyst is impenetrable, immune to unexpected forces and human limitations. When we divert the patient from our tender places, collaborative imagining collapses. There is no room to discuss fantasies of fairy tale reunion, crushing disappointment, paralyzing fears, or unbearable loss. Our patients become careful. They shut down. When we imagine analysts are invulnerable, we do our patients no favors.

The Challenge

I am reminded of the powerful description of intellectual anxiety that emerged when a more traditional analytic practitioner, as he was being wheeled on a stretcher past where his patient sat, worried less about the heart attack he was having and more about how the transference would be contaminated by the breach of the frame.[4] We analysts know no limits to our wish to remain true to the *analytic ideal of anonymity*, part of our analytic constitution – and impossible to uphold. Even when confronted with obvious evidence of our wounds, we hold onto the delusion that scrubbing the frame will protect us from any perception of *actual vulnerability*, an impossible grandiosity.

While never advocating a slipshod frame, incursions, cracks, and surprises are often moments of revelation. Enactments, conflicts in the dyad, or unplanned errors could also be examples of meaning that defy the guardrails of the anonymous identity. In recent years, the presence of illness, violence, racism, political fractures, and the loss of a stable society have affected us all. We do not work in a sealed container, though we may aspire to control interference. Unconscious communications are rarely obedient to conscious directives. Indeed, we rely on this kind of disobedience to expand opportunity in our analytic work. Navigating these instances of incursion, personal, external, and psychic, can facilitate exploration, if the analyst can manage the disruption with understanding and skill. Whether to explore the transference/countertransference dynamic, or understand the subtleties and permeability of the boundary, there are many different meanings that can be derived from the thoughts and actions that emerge. There is much that can be understood in these moments of tension, connection, or breach. But I would argue that inevitably, traces of the analyst's human qualities can be used to facilitate important discussions: the future of the dyad, the impact of external forces, our vulnerability and ultimately, our shared mortality. Such discussions can enrich our work, and their absence may be a consequence of a false belief in analytic restraint as the ultimate gold star.

Over time, it is evident that within our professional community, a technical action may be viewed as an assertion, a demonstration of a professional or theoretical affiliation rather than the result of thoughtful personal reflection. Opinions in our field are strong, no less so regarding self-disclosure. What we do in these instances is often difficult to talk about. And so, ironically, we may remain so guarded about disclosing that we restrict our freedom to talk with each other about what makes self-disclosure so challenging and what it means to each of us. We become fearful of judgment and the loss of our professional network. We fear the presence of our vulnerability as humans will be equated with incompetence as clinicians. But if the analyst's metatheory becomes a bulwark against the anxiety-provoking uncertainty of "what to do" when anonymity is breached, we foreclose one of the most important tenets of our profession: to be curious and open to exploration, even in the most challenging of situations – conditions that challenge us and may require us to ask for help. It has become clearer to me over time, and as I age, that there is a corrosive quality to secrecy – and a sense that, despite efforts to quiet the disclosure, the truth finds a way to sneak out, whatever we hope to conceal.

On this I cannot be sure, but I have come to understand that we can never fully predict how anything may be received or understood by others. There is so much that is unknown and unknowable, even as we seek to explore and discover. I have found that it is better to steer away from the ideas of right and wrong. More useful is how we may think about the subtle nuances that we create in our dyadic spaces, what we can control, and what we cannot, and the impact on our patients of this unusual evolving process. Each of us has entered the analytic world for different reasons. The lopsidedness of the process hints at another truth. We have trouble acknowledging that we learn from our patients, from their disclosures and their complicated knowledge of themselves and of us. They trust us to be helpers in a world of conflict, trauma, and trial, despite the confusion, the injuries, and the risk of intimacy. For their confidence in us, for their agreement to work and live with us in the lopsidedness, I express my gratitude. In truth, life is very personal, and try as we may, there's no way to hide it.

Notes

1 I have found these classic articles regarding therapist anonymity by Jacobs (1999), Gerson (1996), Renik (1999) to be especially valuable to me, but there are many articles on the topic of analyst/therapist self-disclosure that have addressed the dilemmas of the topic.
2 I have written about the essential meaning of this complex process as the resolution of a 'divergent conflict' (Brody, 2016, pp. 138–142) as described by Tony Kris (Kris, 1988, 1990).
3 Brody, S. R. (2013). Entering night country: Reflections on self-disclosure and vulnerability. *Psychoanalytic Dialogues, 23*, 45–58.
4 Arlow (1990).

References

Arlow, J. A. (1990). The analytic attitude in the service of denial. In H. J. Schwartz & A. S. Silver (Eds.), *Illness in the analyst*. Madison, CT: International University Press.
Brody, S. (2013) Entering night country: Reflections on self-disclosure and vulnerability. *Psychoanalytic Dialogues, 23*, 45–58.
Brody, S. (2016). *Entering night country: Psychoanalytic reflections on loss and resilience*. New York: Routledge.
Gerson, S. (1996). Neutrality, resistance, and self-disclosure in an intersubjective psychoanalysis. *Psychoanalytic Dialogues, 6*, 623–645.
Jacobs, T. (1999). On the question of self-disclosure by the analyst: Error or advance in technique. *Psychoanalytic Quarterly, 68*, 159–183.
Kris, A. (1988). Some clinical applications of the distinction between divergent and convergent conflicts. *International Journal of Psychoanalysis, 69*, 431–441.
Kris, A. (1990). Helping patients by analyzing self-criticism. *Journal of the American Psychoanalytic Association, 38*, 605–636.
Renik, O. (1999). Playing with one's cards face up in analysis: An approach to the problem of self-disclosure. *Psychoanalytic Quarterly, 68*, 521–539.
Stern, D. (2020). Field theory and the dream sense: Continuing the comparison of interpersonal/relational theory and Bionian field theory. *Psychoanalytic Dialogues, 30*(5), 538–553.

Section 1

Facing (or Not Facing) the Facts

Introduction to Chapters by H. Housman, R. Deutsch, and J. Schwartz

I suspect that you are reading this book because, in some way, you have been touched by a moment or a time when the personal penetrated the professional. It may be that a very personal event affected you directly, or affected a colleague, or when your own therapist or analyst revealed, or chose not to reveal, an important or even trivial fact. Though I would argue that it is a psychoanalytic illusion that we are ever able to fully maintain a boundary between the personal and the professional, sometimes we are faced with facts that prove especially challenging to manage. There are facts that we might want to reveal, but don't, fearful that our disclosures will compromise a treatment. There are facts that we want to keep private but are unable to conceal because their impact is so significant, or so obvious; there are facts that we may not want to share, but feel we have no choice, as our patients will be affected by our absence or our capacity to attend to them with diligence or focus. There are facts that we choose not to share at all, even though we are affected deeply, and personally.

Issues of privacy play a large part in how or what we decide to share, with our patients and with our colleagues. For some, the analytic dictums that serve to protect the transference through non-disclosure are a great relief when we are faced with a revealing piece of information that we would rather not share with anyone. And these decisions, whether or not to disclose, are very different and deeply personal. Some clinicians have strong feelings and theoretical beliefs about never sharing a vacation destination, while others are comfortable if a patient asks. It may be more challenging if a medical problem or a loss intrudes. It is very hard to share something so personal, something that makes us feel vulnerable and anxious. To me, it is not so much about what we say, or don't say – it's about what we do with the impact of what is disclosed, or not. There are no right or wrong answers.

In the following accounts, you will hear from colleagues who share their experiences as patients and as analysts. Holly Friedman Housman speaks of the seismic impact of the obvious infirmity of her analyst, and his efforts to conceal a serious health issue from her, until he couldn't. She describes the impact on her as a young clinician, and how his actions have impacted her

DOI: 10.4324/9781003584803-2

now, as an experienced clinician. Robin A. Deutsch knew her analyst was ill, but speaks of protecting the dyad, colluding with her analyst, from the imminence of mortality. Writing and publishing an account of her experience led to another personal disclosure and an unfolding of the meaning of self-disclosure to her own patients. Joseph Schwartz shares the loss of an analyst who does disclose, and then the random event that triggers another unexpected disclosure. In each account, we are privileged with first-person descriptions, and the unsettling possibilities when life events intrude on our dyadic space.

In each of these vivid stories, we are given an opportunity to explore the passage of time and the inevitability of loss in the dyad. These are endings that defy the ideals of analytic and psychotherapeutic termination. They caution us to consider the many ways the topic of analyst vulnerability may enter the dyad. It may be useful to wonder how we might anticipate these disruptions and the perceptions of ourselves as human before the fact of it finds its way into the dyad.

1 The Experience of *Non* Self-Disclosure

With a Mortally Ill Analyst

Holly Friedman Housman

When I think about my analyst's tenacity to persevere in his clinical practice despite his illness, I am reminded of Dylan Thomas's well-known poem "Do Not Go Gentle Into That Good Night". For most of the nine months before, during, and after his colon cancer diagnosis my analyst silently, and unbeknownst to me "rage(d) against the dying of the light" (Thomas, 1957).

The death of the long-term and very significant relationship with my analyst was a staggering loss, and, sadly, one for which he did not, or could not, help me prepare. I still have many questions about what got in the way of talking about his illness. Did attachment to his theories of neutrality, abstinence, and anonymity offer protection from self-disclosure, or was it too hard for him to deal with my reaction to his vulnerability while he was trying to contend with his? His classical training asserted that projections and transference had to develop without interference from the analyst's personal reality, in this case, of serious illness, but now I wonder. Would self-disclosure make his illness more real to him? Was he trying to protect me from unnecessary anxiety? Now, an analyst myself, and many years later, I think about Dr. G.'s illness, his return to the office, his subsequent death, and *perhaps his illusion of immortality, which could have been perpetuated by his idea of the analytic process and cure*.

I would like to explore some significant therapeutic decisions, made by my analyst during his illness, and the painful impact his decisions had on me, his analytic patient.

On the Analyst's Inability to Talk About Illness and Death

Dr. G.'s white billowy hair, large sparkling blue eyes, and his handsome presence were striking as he often came rushing into his office suite. He was frequently late and confessed with amusement that he wasn't able to change this about himself, even with an analysis. It was unusual for him to mention anything personal and I was delighted to know something about him. Entering his office, on occasion, felt like venturing into a lion's den. He loomed large as he roared confrontational interpretations in a gruff, but lively, and caring manner: "You're doing a half assed job", or, "maybe you might get around to

DOI: 10.4324/9781003584803-3

thinking more about that". As Red Auerbach, a previous head coach of the Boston Celtics, was known to have said, "You have to know when to kiss them and when to kick them". I felt my analyst seemed to know when to interpret my resistance and defensiveness in a way I thought was humorous and heart-warming. I felt known. He warned me, after hearing various experiences I had with a colleague, that he was a "wolf in sheep's clothing". Although Dr. G. could sound blustery, he conveyed caring, and I felt safe with him.

Dr. G. suggested an analysis after I had worked with him in psychotherapy. After consideration, I began four times per week analysis. The asymmetry of the analytic dyad kept me from knowing a lot about Dr. G. and it was unusual for him to mention anything personal. But there was a lot I did know. I knew every August he vacationed in Wellfleet, on Cape Cod, with his family. I knew the rules: he would charge if I went away when he was working, so I scheduled my vacations to coincide with any days he might be out of the office. Back then, analysts often took the month of August off, so that was when I took my vacation too. I even scheduled my wedding during the month of August so as not to miss sessions with him.

At some point, I learned how many children he had. I was moved after the January 28, 1986 Space Shuttle disaster when Christa McAuliffe, an American teacher, died, and how strongly he responded. He felt she had acted irresponsibly, going up in a space shuttle, taking such a risk, being the mother of two small children. He had five children and felt she had abandoned her two young children with her decision to be part of NASA's Teacher In Space Project. The world was shocked and in mourning, but Dr. G. seemed angry and judged her as an irresponsible parent. His assertion strengthened my experience in the transference that he would protect our work, and that he was committed to me: he would not take any risks, and the treatment would continue until I was ready to terminate.

I hadn't realized that Dr. G. was losing weight until I noticed that his jacket just seemed to hang on him and was no longer filled out by his broad shoulders. I was surprised, and asked him about his weight loss and if he was okay. He brushed away my question and said he was fine. Months later, I asked again about his weight loss, as I could now see his face was gaunt and he appeared to be shrinking in size. Again, he insisted, with a brusque reply, that he was fine. Despite my observation, I didn't connect the dots. I disavowed my thoughts, believed him, and shut out any disturbing thoughts about his health.

I now realize the transference meaning: what was getting replicated in the relationship was my mother's need to protect her privacy and her dismissive reactions to my questions. From an early age I had learned not to ask too many personal questions, since wanting to know more about my mother seemed to annoy her. I assumed she felt shame about having children later in her life, and being, for that time, an older professional mother. When I contained my curiosity, I protected her from embarrassment, and myself from her irritation; though concerned for her discomfort, I felt distanced, shut out, and angry. Dr. G.'s need for privacy intensified the maternal transference, and my dampened curiosity went unanalyzed. My wish to know became repressed and inaccessible to me. As I now write about this, I am reminded of Freud's analytic attitude about his jaw cancer, his prosthesis, and not wanting to be asked about it. My experience was that Dr. G., like Freud, did not want to be asked about his health so I unconsciously (and consciously) complied.

After returning from a weekend away, I retrieved a voice message on my answering machine. I was shaken to hear the voice message of a woman who introduced herself as my analyst's wife. She told me Dr. G. had an emergency hospitalization, and he would contact me when he was ready to return to his office. I was given no information where he was hospitalized, the nature of the medical emergency, his prognosis, or when he was expected to return to his office. Nor was I provided with a phone number should I have any questions or concerns.

In my frantic state, I began calling every hospital in the Boston area asking if Dr. G. had been admitted. This was prior to HIPAA (or the Health Insurance Portability and Accountability Act) going into effect, so I would usually get a response from the person at the hospital. I was totally preoccupied. My husband, acknowledging the gravity of the situation and my determination, took over and transitioned our small children to sleep as I was completely focused elsewhere. In the immediacy of the crisis, and my disbelief, my family fell to the background of my mind as I was struggling to process what I had just heard on the phone. An analyst's illness affects not only the patient but also the patient's entire family.

That my usually sturdy analyst was unreachable seemed unfathomable to me. Without details, my catastrophic fantasies about the emergency hospitalization were unnerving. In my current state of hyperarousal, not knowing Dr. G.'s condition and whereabouts, I felt a profound urgency to locate him. I had a fantasy that he would have wanted to call me himself, but since he couldn't, he would want me to know. Some disclosure of the facts would have given me a better way of dealing with my alarm and would have been enormously useful in helping me regulate and contain my emotional distress, but there was no one to do that with me.

What could I do? My feelings of helplessness and isolation were profound. During the many years I had known him, he had cancelled only three times, informing me of the reason for each. This uncharacteristic abrupt separation began to confuse the way I saw him – sturdy, dependable, infallible, and committed to me and our analytic work. In analysis, we are eventually disabused of our idealizations, but in a way that is optimally disillusioning, not traumatically disillusioning.

I eventually reached Boston's Brigham and Women's Hospital and learned from the Admitting Department that Dr. G. was there and in stable condition. That was the only information I could glean but what did that mean? I immediately sent flowers to the hospital, in the hopes that this small gesture would convey how much he meant to me and how worried and concerned I was about him. In the meantime, I waited.

When Dr. G. returned to the office, two months later, he let me know he had a cancerous tumor that had perforated his colon, necessitating emergency surgery. He thanked me for the flowers and let me know my bouquet was the first he had received. I imagined in the context of my transference dynamic that he understood my feelings of anxiety and sense of urgency to reach him, but he never asked how his absence affected me. Cheerfully, he let me know his doctors told him he was perfectly healthy and cancer free. What joy and what a relief. He was upbeat and looked so much better. His attitude, unfortunately, supported my denial of the seriousness of what had been and what was to come. I wonder now if his cheerful greeting about his health was over-determined, a way to promote a false self for the two of us and reinforce an omnipotent denial of death.

During his absence, I had been talking about my experience with colleagues. Several suggested I terminate treatment with him immediately, but I felt deeply committed to our analytic work, and to him, and I didn't want to – couldn't – simply leave him. I thought these suggestions were odd and that the depth and intensity of my analytic relationship were not understood. I wondered how someone could abandon their therapist at the very time he had cancer. It felt like I was being asked to walk away from an ill family member and I had no intention of doing that. I felt our relationship could withstand whatever emerged. In the analysis, so deeply personal, Dr. G. had conveyed understanding and tolerance for the problematic aspects of me. I was not going to withdraw from him, despite encountering something unthinkable. I naively trusted he would be fine.

I knew Dr. G. as a man who skied some of the most challenging trails in the Northeast – about this he had told me. He projected a persona of strength – not weakness or vulnerability. He embodied masculinity and confidence. In truth we both wanted to deny his fragility, and in our folie à deux, we colluded not to know. As I disavowed concerns about his health, he assured me that he was in perfect health, and I believed him. So, neither one of us discussed his medical condition, other than his bold warning to me "never get colon cancer". He remained guarded and private.

At the end of one session, months after he returned, Dr. G. bellowed out "some people consider their analysts to be their best friends". Taken aback by the intensity of his voice and this statement, I felt confused, guilty; where was this comment coming from, and what did Dr. G. need from me? Of course, he was my best friend, but didn't he know that? I felt immensely grateful for the work we had done together. During the analysis, I started a private practice, fell in love with my husband, got married, we bought a house, and had two children. I believed my emotional growth was the result of our work. Since this was his "door knob" comment at the end of the session, I could only wonder, had I not communicated clearly enough my love and appreciation for him? On that sunny day, as I walked down the back yard path away from his office, I felt upbeat and eager to return the next day to discuss this with him. But that day never came.

I received a call the next day from Dr. G.'s wife saying that he was in the hospital and would be closing his practice immediately; she gave me the contact information for a Dr. W. With my head spinning, I made an appointment. Dr. G. and I had not discussed his current health and there weren't any obvious signals, as there had been previously – no weight loss, or allusions to any other illness or cancer. How could he be in the hospital and suddenly decide overnight to just "close" his practice? There must have been a symptom, a hint of something, yet he never disclosed any facts along the way which could have helped me prepare for this abrupt termination and his impending loss. The call was a total shock.

The Shock of Not Having Been Prepared

How could I say goodbye to my analyst who I knew was alive, but ill, and suddenly not seeing patients? At this juncture there was unwavering hope for some closure. I met with Dr. W., the bridge therapist, or go between, to my analyst, for the sole purpose of wanting to learn more information about Dr. G. "Could Dr. G. maybe have a phone conversation?" I asked. My fantasy was that Dr. G. was surrounding himself with empathic colleagues, who cared about him, and maybe, just maybe, he could make some time for me. I felt tentative asking and a bit guilty about my yearnings. I wondered if I was asking for too much. Would he want to hear from me? It was impossible to make that judgment without more information. What was the reality of his condition?

As Dr. G. was withdrawing, I was feeling cast aside, sidelined, thrown into the deep end. To me, Dr. W. offered some hope of contact, but when I next met with Dr. W., he informed me that a phone call would not be possible. I then considered composing a letter to convey my love and gratitude to Dr. G., which Dr. W. agreed to deliver. During my next visit, I hoped to hear something about Dr. G's response to my letter, but instead, Dr. W. burst into tears letting me know that Dr. G. was dying. The well-kept secret exploded into reality. Death was in the room, and my illusions of my analyst's sturdiness were shattered. His doctors were not going to tell him he would be fine. Dr. W. was distraught, and I was stunned to be with this analyst who I didn't know, now collapsing in front of me. Alongside feelings of confusion and disbelief were feelings of envy. Envious! What an odd feeling at a time like this. But, Dr. W. was given the opportunity to say goodbye, the experience I wanted so desperately for myself. I don't remember now – did he ask me, or did I offer to give a eulogy at the funeral? We agreed on this plan. I was so vulnerable, searching for a way to express my sorrow, deal with my grief, to recognize the significance of our long-term relationship, and to honor Dr. G's memory. My wish to have a role at the funeral and contribute to the reflections about Dr. G's life went unexamined by this consulting analyst, as he too was overwhelmed with his own loss and sadness.

Alone at the Funeral Without a Voice

Writing a eulogy gratified my yearning for the familiarity of my analytic relationship, remembering it, but it was a solitary process. I was isolated, alone, and unable to talk to anyone who knew him. This death occurred long before I was in analytic training, apart from a community of people who knew Dr. G. I anticipated being at a funeral where I would hear about Dr. G. as a real person, meet his family, and be part of a community of mourners trying to navigate their sudden loss. When Dr. W. called to tell me Dr. G. had died, he also told me that the family didn't think it was a wise idea for me to speak at the funeral; Dr. W. informed me he would give the eulogy and quote me, anonymously.

The loss of my role at the funeral presented another whirlwind of raw feelings and again I was left to struggle with them on my own. Not giving the eulogy that I had written, and all that this meant to me felt like an additional trauma. I was angry at Dr. W. for teasing me: offering something, taking it back – a lack of attunement to my pain and wishes. The decision had been made by Dr. G's wife, to protect my confidentiality, but at the time, immersed in the transference, I didn't see that.

Dr. W. didn't ask what part of my eulogy I might want him to read. Instead, he made a decision about what sections he wanted to read. At the funeral, hearing him quote me, without asking my opinion, left me uncomfortably aware of the hypocrisy and seductive role he had played as a bridge analyst. How could he provide a therapeutic holding environment for me during such a profound loss for him? It was another disillusionment. To be referred to an analyst who was also Dr. G's dear friend heightened my unconscious wish that through him, and with him, my relationship with my analyst could be kept alive. But the aftermath of the loss disrupted his capacity to think clearly, to listen to me, and I knew I would never be able to trust him. The illusion of an ongoing connection to Dr. G. through him would always remain. I knew I would not return to his office.

Mourning the Illusion of Immortality in My New Analysis

The relationship had been interrupted, yet I strongly believed Dr. G. would want me to continue my analysis. I missed not only him, but being in analysis. Subsequently, I interviewed five analysts, and chose one I felt best understood my experience. During the treatment, my new analyst, Dr. T., said many times that Dr. G. "was wrong", which initially made me suspicious and confused. At the time, my anger and disappointment with Dr. G. were out of my awareness, a result of deep sadness and a heightened defensive need for idealization. I only became aware of these feelings during this second analysis.

Did Dr. T. really understand me? He was so different from my first analyst.

He was an analyst that challenged the sterile institutional idea of the blank screen. As we analyzed the transference, the relationship deepened, and he helped me to complete the necessary work of mourning. Dr. T., who later became my training analyst, talked openly about his mortality. After our agreed-upon termination, when I returned for "tune up" sessions and I would ask how he was, he would frequently reply with the disarming comment, "I'm still alive". He was a kind human being who had resisted a robotic set of standards. He used to say, after I asked him a personal question, "It's not a state secret, but what do you imagine?" I expected that reaction, encouraging self-reflection, as that is what one does in an analysis. After further exploration he would be forthcoming. I felt Dr. T. listened to me and not to his theory. Before his wife died, he told me, and then took time from his practice. Upon his return he shared with me that he was sad but not depressed. When his sister was dying, Dr. T. let me know he might need to accept a phone call during my analytic hour. He did take the call during my session and openly spoke to his sister's doctor in my presence. This was a radically different way of being together, with the recognition of our shared humanity: people get sick, and we can openly talk about it. When I first interviewed Dr. T. I had asked about his health and he revealed he had had a heart attack many years before, but he was in good health, and took a baby aspirin daily. He assured me that if health issues developed, he would tell me. Initially, these and other demonstrations of his transparency and warmth were unfamiliar, even startling at times, but became reparative for me.

Rage, Rage, Against the Dying of the Light

Many years later, now in a different stage of life, with the emotional separation from my first analyst, I learned through my analytic training about the triumvirate of abstinence, anonymity, and neutrality that were barriers to my knowing the truth about my analyst's final illness. The literature, and the new experience I was having with my second analyst helped me understand what Dr. G. could have given me, but wasn't able to give me, during this traumatic time. I came to learn that most analysts of his generation were influenced by the ideals of transference, resistance, and free association: "the pure gold" of treatment, without much of a nod to external reality. To become accepted as a respected analyst at that time, one had to rigidly adhere to the traditional followers of Freud and Ego Psychology. The unconscious and conscious fears of being an outsider could have brought to the surface what might have been behind my analyst's defensive anonymity. In the American Psychoanalytic Association (APsA), analytic pluralism was then unwelcome, and many felt constrained a fear of being seen as "not analytic enough".

At the time, I understood my analyst's lack of disclosure as his wish for privacy and an analytic effort to direct my curiosity inward. Dr. G's unconscious communication was not to be curious about him, not to ask: "let's get on with the work, we are here to analyze you". This was a familiar family dynamic for me and the reversal of what Sandler refers to as "role responsiveness"

(Sandler, 1976). The irony is that my analyst vacated his empathic role and I found myself in a reversal of our roles – feeling a need to empathize with him.

In retrospect, the paradoxical situation became apparent: it was impossible to do the work when I knew something was wrong. I couldn't talk and I couldn't *not* talk. Dr. G's attempt at anonymity, while non-verbally conveying he was ill, was a contradiction and obstacle to exploring my mind. My analyst projected a false self with his misuse of neutrality, and my task was to see him as a healthy world-class skier. I think how impossible it was to do the work while we were both holding something at bay. The implicit knowing that something was different about him became disavowed in my mind, as I now assume it was in his.

I trusted my analyst to safeguard my emotional well-being. But when his cancer became deadly, he became a victim under siege, unable to safeguard our therapeutic relationship, and me. He was a classical analyst, and that pedagogy nurtured the omnipotent fantasy that analysts were superhumans, God-like, what Ellen Pinsky refers to as an "Olympian delusion" (Pinsky, 2011). This therapeutic stance strengthened a common transference wish: that Dr. G. was immortal and would be here forever, a stance that turned out to be simply wrong, fallacious, and harmful.

During my second analysis, I came to understand what I initially could not put into words: the frame had been broken, and my analyst had abandoned me. I came to recognize, amongst many positive feelings, that I also felt angry, disillusioned, and betrayed. I needed what Winnicott (1960) describes as a good enough "holding environment" (Winnicott, 1960, p. 595) – providing boundaries to the overwhelming intrusion of my fears, and fantasies, which he was unable to do. My second analyst said that Dr. G. "was wrong" about non-disclosure, and I agree with him. But at the same time, I have always felt a deep sense of empathy for him and the obstacles that stood in the way of mourning for both of us. Pinsky reminds us of Cleopatra's confusion about mortality in its literal sense. "When Antony reports to Cleopatra that her rival Fulvia is dead, Cleopatra asks a question we might ask about the psychoanalyst: "Can Fulvia die?" (Pinsky, 2012, p. 30) When Dr. G. told me he had colon cancer, like Cleopatra, I wondered if Dr. G. could die. His mortality was obscured by my denial and supported by his.

When Dr. G's wife called me the second time, I couldn't comprehend how Dr. G. could suddenly be too ill to continue with his practice. Just hours before, he had been sitting behind the couch and talking to me. There were so many thoughts and feelings I wanted to share with him, and I felt the loss of a termination phase for each of us. During our brief phone call, Dr. G's wife's tone was business-like and I felt I had become nothing more than a name to cross off on her to-do list. But at that moment, I also felt a bond with her, sharing this impending loss and her own grief and sadness. As a caretaker too, I wanted to protect her by not asking questions and interfering with her awful task, the bearer of this disturbing news to my analytic siblings. I realized I didn't even know the name of the woman who followed my analytic hour.

Just her warm familiar face. We always said hello when I left the office. She too would be on the list.

How different the experience would have been if, after his return from colon cancer surgery, Dr. G. and I had discussed reality, and my fears about confronting my own mortality, his mortality, separation, and impending loss. Then we would have also had the intersubjective acceptance to talk about my fantasies, transference reactions, and what he may have wanted to say to me, while still maintaining the analytic attitude. I remain haunted by the question of how much was in his awareness.

A Friend Has Led the Way: Acknowledging Mortality

Lauren, who died many years after my analyst, offers the ideal of what I wish my analyst could have done for me. My colleague, and close friend, Lauren accepted living with cancer throughout her illness, and subsequent death. She faced this immensely challenging personal situation with determination, curiosity, and dignity. She was courageous and ethical. How she handled her illness, and death continues to affect me.

When Lauren was diagnosed with pancreatic cancer, and before her surgery, she informed her patients and colleagues about her medical condition. Her acceptance allowed her to prepare her family, patients, colleagues, and friends for her loss. She was a role model and an inspiration for how to help those she cared about, and those who cared about her, to say goodbye. Sometimes she would ask her patients, "how is my illness affecting you?" Before her surgery, she prearranged with patients that she would be away from her practice for a certain length of time. She told her patients that she would be undergoing a series of chemotherapy after her surgery and their appointments might need to be rescheduled when she returned to the office.

Two years after Lauren's initial surgery (a Whipple procedure), when she learned her cancer had recurred, she started a termination process with her patients. She was quite forthcoming about her cancer, her impending death, and asked each one of them if they wanted to be notified after her death. Lauren was straightforward with her patients, but how much she disclosed depended on each patient's diagnosis, length of treatment, and their need to know. She took her time, sought out consultations concerning her clinical terminations, and discussed her illness in her peer groups; Lauren wore a wig, lost weight, and acknowledged with her patients how her health and appearance were changing. She remained unusually open to questions, exploring fantasies and affect, while providing information.

Lauren was not only thoughtful and compassionate in her care for her patients but also considerate and generous with those she appointed to execute her wishes. I had the privilege of being one of the three people who were assigned as an executor of her professional will as she believed it would be unfair to ask one person to manage the strain of this task. Lauren allocated money in her Professional Will to reimburse each of us for the consultations she wanted us to have with her patients. We, her Executors, were deeply moved by her confidence in us to carry out her well-thought-out plans for her patients, and generosity to each of us after she died. Lauren thought about which one of us would contact each patient, and each was invited to the memorial service. She wanted them to know that their attendance was welcomed. Rather than being isolated with this sad task, the three of us had each other to talk to about our contacts with her patients, and the impact this had on our own grieving process. The initial contact with Lauren's patients was a bit intricate after her death. We were reluctant to leave detailed voice messages: some people were hard to reach. Others didn't return our initial calls. Each patient had different needs that ranged from detailed questions about her death, to not asking questions, to wanting to talk about the memorial service, or wanting to make an appointment with one of us, to grieve. Some were satisfied with simply the initial phone contact and thanked us for calling. With Lauren's patients, no one requested a referral for ongoing therapy since Lauren addressed this with each of her patients during the termination process. However, if there had been a sudden death, and Lauren hadn't made a referral, we would have regarded this as our Executor role.

Lauren's therapeutic endings pay homage to the dignity and love she afforded to each unique and special person in her practice and in her community. I recall how Lauren found such strength in maintaining her humanity in the face of adversity. How she dealt with her mortality was remarkable. Yet, even Lauren had an overarching omnipotent wish to defend against her helplessness. Feeling so out of control with her perilous cancer, she needed to be in control of disseminating her personal information. Lauren had a well-respected and honored need to be the voice that clearly directed who was told and what they were told.

Each summer the Boston Symphony Orchestra performs Beethoven's Ninth for the last concert of the summer season. I have fond memories of picnicking on the lawn at Tanglewood with my friend and hearing the passionate orchestra and chorus, listening to the Ode to Joy,

> *Whom the crown of stars doth honor,*
> *Whom the hymns of Seraphs bless,*
> *To the goodly Soul this glass*
> *O'er the tent of stars up yonder!*
>
> (Schiller, 1786)

and feeling the bittersweet ending of the season together. Now, six years after Lauren's death, I continue to imagine sitting on the lawn at Tanglewood during this last concert and metaphorically raising a toast to her for her clinical judgment, receptivity, therapeutic transparency, courage, and her humanity, which allowed her patients to talk with her about their panoply of feelings during a complicated mourning process. As I write about Lauren navigating her illness with such care for her patients and friends, I hope, when I am faced with my mortality, I can model her compassion and openness while experiencing such intense vulnerability as Lauren so beautifully taught me.

I was reminded of Lauren and my second analyst's openness when my husband had a recent hospitalization. While I was waiting for a call from his doctor, I let my patients know there might be an interruption and why. Having internalized the values of Lauren and Dr. T. helped me recognize what I wanted to do and what some patients might need from me. If some patients were concerned about the impact my husband's illness was having on me, and in turn the impact it was having on them, we could talk about it. I want to be an analyst who conveys an analytic attitude that allows for this kind of openness.

Increasingly we acknowledge that dependable, consistent, and intense relationships can abruptly change. This is a disorienting and traumatic dislocation to patients, their analysts, and their colleagues. The COVID pandemic made us aware that we were all vulnerable to a virus that could be transmitted in the office. Our mortality entered our therapeutic conversations as our precautions shifted our practices. The pandemic, my friend's courage, my first analyst's denial, and my second analyst's openness, all profoundly affected my capacity for transparency with my patients and how we might do better in the face of these very human challenges.

Practical Considerations: A Way Forward

It has been 30 years since my analyst's death. Now, I hold a leadership role at the Boston Psychoanalytic Society and Institute (BPSI) and have come to recognize that our analytic institutes can do better to protect patients and candidates as we are aging. We need to have a radical openness to acknowledging our vulnerability and mortality, our own, as well as our colleagues. We need to teach ideas about self-disclosure: when to disclose, how to disclose, to which patients to disclose, which patients not to disclose to, and why not. We need to promote open discussions about self-disclosure through courses, case presentations, academic lectures, discussion groups, supervision, and looking at our growing literature on this subject. Our psychoanalytic culture needs this radical shift. The leadership at each institute, beginning with the Board of Trustees, must endorse this effort for any change to take place.

Safeguarding our patients' continuity of care needs to begin when we start our practices. This is an opportune time to do a Professional Will as part of establishing one's practice, seamless from the beginning. Just as we think about who will cover our practice while we are away, another necessary question to consider is who will contact our patients if something should happen to us. This is simply good medical ethics. A professional license, professional and office insurance are requirements that safeguard our practices and our patients.

I have a Professional Will. I have asked three members of my peer consultation group to function in this therapeutic role for me and contact the people who would be directly impacted should something unexpected occur. Patients would receive a phone message with a request to contact them, not a note left on an office door. Although still unsettling, patients would be given the opportunity to absorb the information about my health with a predesignated, experienced colleague. They would not have to process the shock alone.

The BPSI Board of Trustees supports the value of Professional Wills for our trainees and graduate members. We have entrusted our Education Committee to explore options and offer recommendations about BPSI's position on this issue with its members. It seems likely that we will develop a process in which members are invited to submit the names of two colleagues who have agreed to provide continuity of care to the member's patients and supervisees in the event of incapacity. We also offer Professional Will templates on our website, inviting our members to utilize them as they consider crafting their own more expansive Professional Will. I anticipate our Ethics Education Committee will continue to provide a forum for ongoing discussions of ethical standards regarding the closure of our practices, due to illness, sudden death, or retirement, and will continue to consult with members about creating a Professional Will. The leadership at BPSI has recognized the necessity of planning for the continuity of care for our patients and trainees, and by doing so, we are taking better care of our professional selves and our families. We will all become the beneficiaries.

Closing Thoughts

We all want to protect our patients from any sudden trauma. While writing this chapter, so many conflicting feelings arose once again – feelings that I thought had been laid to rest. Even now, I think about the analytic culture of anonymity that my analyst was practicing while struggling with a body that was defeating him. I still feel heartbroken for him, his other patients, and for me. I imagine the conflicting feelings Dr. G. must have experienced while he was ill and wanted so much to be able to continue to work. What a tragedy for my analyst to experience such a premature closure. But even his death he has taught me so much about caring for others, and I remain indebted to him for what he has taught me through his own vulnerability.

References

Beethoven, L. van. Symphony No. 9 in D Minor, Op. 125 (with the choral finale, "Ode to Joy," featuring the text by Friedrich Schiller, 1786).

Pinsky, E. (2011). The Olympian delusion. *Journal of the American Psychoanalytic Association, 59*, 351–375.

Pinsky, E. (2012). Physic himself must fade: A view of the therapeutic offering through the lens of mortality. *American Imago, 69*, 29–56.

Sandler, J. (1976). Countertransference and role responsiveness. *International Review of Psycho-Analysis, 3*, 43–47.

Thomas, D. (1957). *The collected poems of Dylan Thomas*. New York: New Directions Publishing Corporation.
Winnicott, D. W. (1960). The theory of the parent-infant relationship. *International Journal of Psychoanalysis, 41*, 585–595.

Acknowledgment

I would like to thank Stephen Bernstein and Andrea Celenza for their invaluable suggestions in the development of this chapter.

2 So Very Human

Reality's Messy Intrusion and Self-Disclosure

Robin A. Deutsch

In 2005, surprisingly to me, my analyst died while she was away on vacation. I published a paper (Deutsch, 2011) about my experience of digesting the impact of her sudden loss. In that paper, I disclosed, in the form of reported dreams and my interpretation of them, an intimate view of my psychological state at the time of that loss. Some years later (2017), I presented a paper on what I believed I had been disclosing in writing about my reaction to my analyst's death. In that paper, I explored that disclosure from the vantage points of being a patient, of being an analyst, and of being an author who exposed her experience of this impactful loss.

In this essay, I intend to review how these events have affected me as an analyst and what I have come to believe about managing disclosure of personal events in the context of my professional life. I am not making recommendations or rules about what analysts should do. Rather I am reflecting on my experience and what I've done with that reflection, as I've integrated the impact of the loss of my analyst from an undisclosed illness combined with my experience of disclosing that impact publicly. I also wish to reflect on the importance of being able and willing to use our disclosures to our patients in the service of the treatment itself. With this essay, I am inviting each reader to immerse themselves in the messiness of life, its impact on how each of us practices analysis, and how we find our way with our patients.

As a group, analysts and therapists prefer to think of ourselves as managing the impact of life's events better than other humans. We believe we will be able to go to the office and help our patients with the same equanimity every day; that we will know if we are off kilter in some way that interferes with our regular ability to work. While we simultaneously know this isn't true, as we seem to know it for other analysts, it remains harder to assess for ourselves. We prefer the illusion that what impacts us is controlled in its effects on our patients; and that all of those messy events do not trickle down to our patients. It is hard for us to keep in mind that our patients are not immune when we experience great personal stress. We need to be willing to help our patients deal with our stress as it reverberates in the office.

After my analyst's death, I discovered that she had struggled for over two decades with a health problem which, from the beginning, was known to be

DOI: 10.4324/9781003584803-4

terminal. Despite evidence of her illness in the office, I did not ask. It was only after a colleague eventually told me that my analyst was going to die that I asked my analyst what was wrong. Even when I inquired, her response came with minimal elaboration, and some reassurance that her illness was not following a predictable trajectory, hinting that the diagnosis was in question. Looking back, she was essentially denying the progressive nature and inevitable outcome of her illness. I did not press her for more information.

The statement I made that she died without warning was not precisely the case. To be clear, her death occurred while she was away and planned to return. I have come to understand that I did not want to put the pieces together. I do not fault either of us for being human. The way in which each of us handled this event has impacted how I manage disclosures about myself when it comes, what to disclose, when, and how.

The last three months of my analyst's life have most informed my clinical practice. During this time, everything with her and in the office felt wrong. I commented in every session about how wrong things felt. A month before her death, my analyst disclosed that I was right; she was not herself but said reassuringly that she was with me still. While I found this comment reassuring, the climate continued to feel off. Her usual curiosity and engagement were missing. On the day before we were to resume after the holiday break, I got a phone call from a colleague, informing me that my analyst had died during the night. I never got to say goodbye. As it turned out, our jointly constructed relationship to her health foreclosed my opportunity to say goodbye to her while she was still alive. While I believe I benefitted from this construction in many ways, I felt betrayed by being denied the opportunity to know and to say goodbye.

The First Disclosure

The original article that I wrote about the impact of my analyst's death is an intensely personal document in which I used my dreams as data to describe how I terminated my analysis with my then analyst, mourned and moved forward in my life. Like a photograph, it immerses the reader in my psyche in a singular moment of time. In my earliest dreams, I made my dream analyst disclose to me what she had in fact not disclosed in real life: that she was terminally ill and that her death was near. I made her tell me in dreamlife that which she was, in reality, unable to tell me. I offer three dreams here to give the reader an example of the nature of my 2011 disclosure:

Dream 1. My analyst tells me she is going to close her practice in two months.

Dream 2. My analyst tells me she is too tired to go on. She says we can talk about it if I want.

Dream 3. I am in my analyst's office. When I come in, she tells me she is dying and asks if I want to know what is wrong. I say yes. She is sitting on one end of her couch, and I, on the other. As she sits on the couch and reads to me about her illness from a book – she begins to cry. I do as well. She asks if I am all right. I say I am fine and reach to hold her hand as we cry together.

Each dream in the original paper is annotated by my understanding of my mourning process. My emotional life at that time was there for anyone to read.

In retrospect, it is not just the distress at the loss of my analyst that I am disclosing, but by using my dreams, I have disclosed my conscious and unconscious reactions to her death, my intense attachment to her and the depth of my loss and mourning.

In the 2017 essay, I take up the impact of my disclosures on my patients in the original 2011 essay (Deutsch, 2017). At the time, writing helped me express what I felt inexpressible: reconnecting with my analyst, processing her death, and terminating my analysis. I was not fully aware of what I was disclosing in writing, but more importantly, I did not think about the potential reader's reaction to the paper. I certainly wasn't thinking about what current or future patients might think of me if they read it. At several points in the 2011 essay, I report how I protected my analyst, and myself from my knowing and worrying about her health while she was alive, in this way protecting her against how angry and betrayed I might have felt if I had let myself know how seriously ill she was. As I go on to describe my struggle to enter a relationship with a new analyst, fears of betrayal, disloyalty, and guilt about continuing to survive, about having a more fulfilling life in the face of her death, are prominent. But even more, I disclosed that I am a human who can close my mind to reality. This awareness helped me consider how disclosure of such humanness impacts a treatment, and how this humanness is absorbed by my patients.

The Evolution of a Disclosure in the Dyad

Samuel, an only child from a family with significant emotional, social, and financial impoverishment, has read my paper and bought my book. He has never had very much to say about his reactions to my disclosure of these experiences, and even with encouragement, would often find himself tongue-tied and silent for large parts of his hour. He has continued to fall silent or become confused when his awareness of his attachment to me is more alive. Beginning shortly after he reported having read my paper, Samuel has periodically voiced the fear that he will lose me before the end of his analysis. My vacation sets off worries I will not return. Over time, he has expressed this anxiety but hasn't understood why this idea would come to mind. Why he might be thinking about this has been limited by his chronic inability to allow his thoughts free rein. For several years, he has put forth the idea that he will run out of money, need to move away, or perhaps take a job that will interfere with his sessions. At those moments, he is unable to keep in mind that we have altered his schedule more than once over the years based on his needs, or that I have been willing to adjust his fee based on his finances.

I have often wondered if reading my paper has made him worry that I will die prematurely as my analyst did. Each time his worry has appeared, we have tried to better understand it, but I believe his fear of knowing what he thinks has kept a lid on his fully thinking about this idea. As the result of his analysis, Samuel has made a fair amount of progress in remaining present and in emotional contact with me during sessions. It is progress that I think both of us can feel proud of.

During this time, Samuel arrived for an appointment in a tumultuous state, worried that I wouldn't be in the office for his appointment. When I commented about his constant fearfulness that he will lose me, he responded that he is always afraid of this. "I suppose at some point I will stop seeing you, but when that will be and how far along I will be in my development, I don't know".

I press him. "What are the circumstances under which we would stop?"

He demurs, but now we are in a place where I can continue to press. I suggest that I believe he does have fantasies about how we come to an end.

Much to my surprise, he says, "You'll retire. I end up working in a job that means I can't meet with you any longer".

Saying that something might happen to me that would impact him, is more revealing of his internal anxieties than usual.

For the first time, in response, I say, "I know you read my paper. I know you know my analyst died, and since that time, you have periodically voiced concern that something would interfere with your completing your analysis with me. I can't help but wonder how reading my paper has impacted you in our work together". I continue: "You've never really said much about reading my paper".

He is surprised and unaware that he began to voice his worry over losing me after he read my paper. He says he can't remember that much, and when I point out that he remembers some things, he says, "You mean that your analyst died? I wonder if that will happen to me". He goes on. "Maybe I'm thinking that I took the fear of your death, or of losing you, as a trigger for anxiety about going forward. Thinking about your analyst's death or your possible death told me that I was more attached to you than I would have thought. I didn't want to know all of this, so I forgot".

I wonder if I have forced Samuel to know something he wasn't quite ready for. I say, "Maybe you feel I overexposed myself in my article".

"Maybe", Samuel allows. "Not that you shouldn't have, but that *I* couldn't commit myself to writing. . . . I'm worried I might learn something about you that I don't want to know. I am afraid I will find something in your article that leads me to fear you are dying. I don't want to know how much you mean to me these days, to be explicit".

He becomes confused and confusing.

I add, "You don't want to say something as directly as you are thinking it".

Samuel begins to talk about mourning: "I'm worried that I might start thinking about letting you go when I've just begun to get connected to you".

We finish out the hour with the following exchange.

I say: "You would see something in my relationship to my analyst that would come to feel unbearable to you".

In response, Samuel says, "Yes. I might find something in my relationship with you . . . something I don't want to know. I'm not sure where to put that fear because I'm blaming the article".

After a silence, Samuel continues "I had a thought – but lost it".

I reply, "You lost your thought after blaming the article. I wrote the article, I agreed to publish it. Would it be the article or me that you want to blame?"

Surprisingly, Samuel adds, "I think it would be me. I decided to expose myself to a relationship with you. Even though I chose to enter a relationship with you, my illusion of absolute control hasn't dissipated. How I control it is by not letting myself remember the article".

This was the end of the hour. At that moment, we have used my disclosures to understand more about Samuel's internal life and his apprehensions about connection.

A Different Time – A Different Disclosure

Several years ago, my husband had an emergency hospitalization. To be at the hospital with him, I called my patients, telling them I had a family emergency and that I would return to the office the following week. However, as the end of the week was approaching, the discharge date remained uncertain, so once again I called my patients and delayed my return; I told them I would be in the office the following week but would call to confirm my return. Upon my return, my patients were curious, worried for me, and not surprisingly for themselves; my absence had triggered not just reality concerns, but childhood experiences of abandonment and unreliability. During this first week back at work, patients expressed their worries and had many ideas about what my absence from work meant to them and to me. I decided to offer a choice: if they felt they needed to know more, I would tell them. For those patients who wanted to know, I disclosed that my husband had been hospitalized and was recovering. I revealed no further information. I did not tell those patients who said they did not want to know. Reflections of my experience with my analyst contributed to this compromise. I felt it was an undue burden to ask patients to digest an unexplained and sudden absence without being willing to offer them a choice about knowing more, but only should they wish. Neither did I wish to deny people the opportunity to know more if they felt it would help them manage their worries about me, nor did I wish to burden people with this knowledge, if they felt they did not want to know. About half of my practice wished to know more, and the other half wished no further information. Of course, I took this path knowing that, whatever each person decided, at some point I would need to be willing to discuss my decisions and my actions, when my patient was ready.

When my husband was readmitted to the hospital just a week later for life-threatening side effects related to the treatment, I again canceled appointments. For those who knew, I indicated that my husband was re-hospitalized. For those who didn't know or didn't want to know, I merely said I needed to be out of the office again. After his discharge, I remained out of the office to organize at-home care, planning to return to work after a previously scheduled ten-day vacation. One month after his initial hospitalization, and at the beginning of my planned vacation, my husband died. When I returned to the office ten days later, some asked about him immediately, while others didn't ask again for a few weeks. Now, I was faced with the dilemma of how, or in what way, to disclose his death. For those who asked me directly how he was doing, I said that I was sorry to tell them that he had died. For people who didn't ask, I said nothing.

By disclosing his death, I had injected my real loss into the consulting room. It soon became clear that some of the people who knew were reluctant to share concerns about their own lives. I pressed them about their reticence. Was their experience of me different? If so, how? Did I appear fragile? Were they worried about my resilience? In what way? One patient, in treatment to explore his dating relationships after becoming a widower a few years prior, now had little to say about himself. For several weeks after my return, this previously engaged and talkative man with an active dating life seemed to have nothing particular to talk about. He wondered about discontinuing treatment. I explored what he thought about having so little to say. I suggested that because he knew of my husband's death, and that we now shared the state of widowhood, it was challenging to tell me about the forward progression in his life, when mine had hit a massive snag. This man, who often felt responsible for other's feelings, agreed that he had to be there for me, and to take care of me. I said to him that while I appreciated his sentiment, this would be a reversal of our roles and my misuse of him and his treatment. This relatively small intervention seemed to free him to think of himself again, and the familiar rhythm of our work together returned shortly. In addition, it gave us a window into understanding more about his feelings of duty, responsibility, and sacrifice toward others at his own expense.

For those who preferred not to know, the issue also appeared. This group consisted of people who held me at arm's length and seemed, at least on the surface, to allow themselves very little curiosity about me. For these individuals, I came to believe that any disclosure I might make would require them to take responsibility for my well-being, often a historical remnant from their family of origin. However, this transference manifestation wasn't available to be discussed at the time because these were individuals, unlike the dutiful patient described earlier, who were not yet able to have that intimate a dialogue.

One year later, I decided to tell everyone that I would be out for hip replacement surgery. Although messy, simply stating that I would be away for six weeks felt inadequate, leaving them to wonder about my health and sturdiness, without the opportunity to address their concerns. In deciding how much to disclose, I weighed each patient's past preference for information against the likelihood that they might wrongly connect this absence to my previous one. Both times previously, I had been unavailable to them, and had different privacy considerations. In this case, I was balancing the risk of unwanted intrusion against the potential anxiety of an unarticulated abandonment. Furthermore, I felt it was more advisable for me to be transparent about my surgery in the very unlikely circumstance of an untoward surgical outcome. This pending absence gave me the opportunity to remind them that, previously, they had not wanted information, but that this time I had not given them a choice. I wondered about their reaction to my intrusive disclosure, and the opportunity to prepare and talk with me as they prepared for my absence.

Conclusion

There is no getting away from it. Life is messy and an analyst's life is no exception. Analytic writers have been wrestling with this messiness for decades, often promoting a rule that not disclosing is protecting the patient and the analysis. From Abend (1982) to Gerson (1996) to Zemmelman (2017), what, how much and why to disclose has been broadly theorized, described, and debated. Rosner (1986) speculated that the trend at the time to treat the analyst's absence due to illness, no matter how serious that illness might be, as any other separation, for him brought into focus the conflict between what is humane and what might arguably be best technically. He stated, "Honesty and truthfulness are part of the countertransference, as are fear, withholding, anxiety, and subterfuge. The assumption that an analyst's conflicts can be hidden from the patient's unconscious is a fiction" (Rosner, 1986, p. 365). Hart (2022), writing 36 years after Rosner (1986), states, "Ultimately, the idea of neutrality forces us to the limits of our collective wishful fantasy that the psychoanalytic process could ideally be exclusively about and for the patient" (Hart, 2022, p. 346).

It has been my objective to broaden the discussion about analyst disclosure beyond the conventional. I have described the circumstances that influenced my ideas about analyst disclosure as well as how I have worked clinically with my disclosures to understand and help my patients understand, not just the impact of my intrusions, but more about themselves. I also have drawn attention to how I elected to balance the conflict between my need for personal privacy and the potential impact of my privacy on my patient.

This essay, which focuses on the ways in which my relationship to analyst self-disclosure has evolved is, in and of itself, full of disclosures for the reader to find. I have disclosed my belief in the importance of not backing away from how our patients know us. More specifically, I am suggesting that there is something important about revealing our humanness in the clinical encounter and our willingness to contend with this humanness as its impact is felt by our patients. I believe that we must be willing to encourage and at times to push our patients to wrestle with their reactions to our disclosures, not just inside themselves but with us as well.

These thoughts have brought me full circle back to my invitation to consider the impact of self-disclosure in the analytic setting. I believe that I have become more fluid in disclosing facts about reality intrusions for two main reasons: I have first-hand experience of what it means to a patient not to know, and because I feel more able to help my patients with their reactions to knowing. While the frame is generally protective, it can also stifle. I am more comfortable stepping beyond our rules and am more willing to deal with the consequences of my disclosures. I would suggest that by not attending to or welcoming our patients' reactions to our inevitable intrusions into the analytic process, intentional or inadvertent, our patients are deprived of recognizing the humanness in us; and we are deprived of knowing that, in revealing our humanness to our patients, we offer something important to them.

Bibliography

Abend, S. M. (1982). Serious illness in the analyst: Countertransference considerations. *Journal of the American Psychoanalytic Association, 30,* 365–645.

Deutsch, R. A. (2011). A voice lost, a voice found: After the death of the analyst. *Psychoanalytic Inquiry, 31,* 526–535.

Deutsch, R. A. (2017). *Doubling disclosure: Disclosures' hall of mirrors*. Paper Presented at the American Psychoanalytic Association Meetings, New York.

Gerson, S. (1996). Neutrality, resistance, and self-disclosure in an intersubjective psychoanalysis. *Psychoanalytic Dialogues, 6,* 623–645.

Hart, A. (2022). Neutrality as a 'white lie': Discussion of Gabbard, Holmes, and Portuguese. *Journal of the American Psychoanalytic Association, 70,* 335–349.

Rosner, S. (1986). The seriously ill or dying analyst and the limits of neutrality. *Psychoanalytic Psychology, 3,* 357–371.

Zemmelman, S. (2017). Just this side of the edge: Clinical perspectives in the face of serious illness and death of the analyst. *Jung Journal, 11*(1), 35–46. https://doi.org/10.1080/19342039.2017.1262667

3 Self-Disclosure, Mortality, and What Comes Next

Joseph Schwartz

This essay was occasioned by an invitation to offer brief comments at the ongoing Discussion Group on Self-Disclosure at the APsaA meetings held in 2022 in Boston. We were still in the throes of COVID and there was palpable anxiety shot through the experience. Not coincidentally, this iteration of this long-standing Discussion Group brought together issues of self-disclosure and mortality in the psychoanalytic experience. Our presenter, Linda Emmanuel, had been instrumental in forming an ongoing discussion group exploring the ways that experiences of mortality in our patients get understood and processed in analytic treatments. In the spirit of the open-ended invitation to contribute some thoughts to the conversation at the Self-Disclosure Discussion Group, I did not focus on Linda Emmanuel's presentation, but offered my experience of being the patient who received self-disclosures related to my analyst's unforeseen and, ultimately, tragic engagements with mortality.[1]

It is worth taking a moment to unpack what we mean by self-disclosure. Since the publication of Irwin Hoffman's paper "The Patient as Interpreter of the Analyst's Experience" (Hoffman, 1983), we can no longer maintain the epistemological blank screen posture of analytic anonymity. We are revealing things about ourselves all the time, and we invariably offer our patients a stimulus-rich environment. We speak with a particular accent and timbre; sometimes we have a cold; we laugh at some things but not at others; we have decorated our offices according to our functional and aesthetic preferences; and on and on. And the presumption that our patients are not drawing inferences, often disconcertingly accurate inferences, from the wealth of incidental information we provide, is no longer tenable. But this is not generally what we mean by self-disclosure. And over the past 85 years, since Paula Heimann (1950) and Annie Reich (1951) articulated very different understandings of the origins and uses to be made of countertransference experience, the analytic literature has been brimming with argumentation regarding the issues they first engaged. Certainly, some of the ways psychoanalysts have chosen to make their countertransference experience available to their patients come closer to what we mean by self-disclosure. I have in mind, for example, (there are many, many others) papers by Christopher Bollas (1983), and Jody Davies (1994, 1999), very carefully argued instances of the active use of countertransference

DOI: 10.4324/9781003584803-5

that involve a version of self-disclosure. But then there are occasions when we as analysts and psychoanalytic psychotherapists explicitly share something of our personal history or circumstances, sometimes by necessity, sometimes by choice, that are very clearly acts of self-disclosure that throw away any pretense of maintaining anonymity and yet still maintain the discipline of careful analytic work with the best interests of analysands still foremost in mind (cf. Hoffman, 1996). And who among us hasn't shared a personal vignette to illustrate and personalize a moment in psychotherapeutic engagement in the hope of maximizing therapeutic impact? Cautionary voices have been raised about the increasing freedom some analysts have felt that might make their own experience too central to the analytic encounter (Slochower, 2017).

I turn now to the first of the two instances in which I was the recipient of analytic self-disclosure that I will discuss. About six months into my first training analysis, my analyst announced that he would be taking six weeks off to recuperate from upcoming coronary bypass surgery. He offered this in a fairly matter-of-fact manner. He gave me the name of a colleague I had never met (a very close friend of his as it happened) to whom I could reach out should anything of significance or urgency come up for me during his absence. This was clearly a surgery that was necessary, but planned well in advance. It was not an emergency. It was evident that he fully expected the surgery to be successful and that we would resume my analysis upon his return. I was certainly free to voice whatever anxieties I may have had about the seriousness of his medical situation as I was free to talk about anything else that happened to be on my mind. I imagine I did so in passing, knowing my characterological reluctance to create conflict, cause distress, ruffle feathers that I imagine I felt did not need any further ruffling from me. As it turned out, the surgery was successful, but the patient subsequently died. Twenty-four hours after the surgery, my analyst had a fatal cardiovascular event, something I found out from my then wife, who received a call from a representative of the institute to let me know that my analyst had died. It was a very different time and to call the atmosphere at the institute austere might itself be generous. But for the thoughtfulness and concern of one of the training analysts who had interviewed me as an applicant, I was left to sort this out on my own. But the focus here is on self-disclosure. In an even earlier psychoanalytic era, even this self-disclosure might have been seen as offering too much information. Why not simply say "I will be away from my practice for the next six weeks", and allow me as analysand to fantasize about what might be transpiring uncontaminated by his external realities? Thankfully I was not put in that absurd position. But what are our responsibilities once such a disclosure has been offered? How energetically are we to pursue the impact of that disclosure? In this instance, I suspect that the two of us colluded in avoiding substantive exploration of the seriousness of his medical condition. After all, what did it mean that I was given the name of a very close personal friend and colleague as covering person? This would only make sense if he was not entertaining seriously the possibility of not surviving this medical crisis. Could I have been expected to discuss the full range of my feelings, loss and sadness to be sure, but also anger, with someone who himself would be dealing with his own profound grief and loss? My point here is not what exactly my analyst should or should not have told me about the particulars of his health status but rather what was required once he did so in whichever way he believed to be psychoanalytically sound. Rather, I think that our responsibility requires us to more actively pursue the impact of such a disclosure, not simply to allow associations to reveal that impact, especially when heightened personal anxieties on both the analysand's and the *analyst's* part are likely in play, something that most of us on the couch would at least preconsciously intuit would be the case. I don't know how I would have responded to such an active invitation had one been offered, but the psychoanalytic technique of that bygone era would certainly have proscribed that departure from abstinence and neutrality. Let's wait and see what comes up was the order of the day.

I turn now to a far denser and more complex disclosure. Several years later, now well into my second training analysis, I came into work at McLean Hospital to find one of our secretaries quietly crying at her desk. I sat down with her and learned that her eldest granddaughter had just been diagnosed with leukemia. I, myself, had had an older cousin die of leukemia when he was 15 years old, and I was 12. Memories from that time in my childhood were on my mind in my analytic hours that week: the impact that my cousin's death had on his two-years-younger brother and parents; the absence of any discussion with me or my cousins of what was transpiring during the year and a half of his illness; and the horrifying impact that the first generation of chemotherapy agents had on him. Seemingly out of nowhere, my analyst said, "You've probably heard that there's a serious illness in my family". I was stunned. I had no idea what he was talking about. He didn't go into details. He clearly thought that I was alluding to an awareness of a painful matter that I was, in a roundabout way through the material I had been offering, trying to broach. I should be clear that had I known that there was such an illness in his family I would indeed have had a very difficult time bringing it up directly. His understanding of my characteristic tendency toward avoidance certainly provided some basis for wondering whether I was in internal tension around such a painful, tender issue and needed some help in broaching it. Thankfully, he did not insist that I knew more about his circumstances than I actually did. This moment occurred as my negative transference was in full flower organized around my sense of the remoteness that was an outgrowth of his classical psychoanalytic technique from which this startling self-disclosure was such a singular departure. We carried on as if nothing unusual, not to say cataclysmic, had transpired. Some months later, I received a call from my analyst telling me that his youngest son had died and that he would be taking a week off and that we would resume our work together when he returned. I did attend the memorial service that was held for his son, and this allowed for a deepening of my appreciation of the enormity of his loss and a growing empathy and warmth for him.

Nonetheless, I do know from my own experience that this self-disclosure and the intrusion of a painful reality from my analyst's life occluded much necessary analytic work on my part for the remaining several years I remained in treatment. That is not to say that my analysis ground completely to a halt, but there was for me a kind of mild dissociation and avoidance around the expression of any criticism, anger, or dissatisfaction and that this remained unaddressed by either of us. There was simply no way, or at least no way that we found, to work with and through the painful reality that sat between us. It was surely not a coincidence that the birth of my second child, my son, was the external event that set the termination date for my analysis, though I am quite certain that neither of us made the connection to the death of his own son explicit. I don't pretend to know how I would have managed work with my own patients were I ever to find myself trying to do the work we do while my own young adult child was going through an illness that I knew would end in death. But that does not obviate our obligation to try as best as we can to prevent the therapeutic space from constricting.

But let's imagine for a moment that I had been out sick the day that our part-time secretary was in the office crying and that my analytic hours had taken their usual course with no external event precipitating the memories of my cousin's death from leukemia. It is likely that I would have continued pummeling my analyst with my complaints about his long silences that I experienced as distance, disengagement, and a reluctance to mix it up with me with all its attendant transferential implications. He would likely not have said anything about his son's illness until I received a call from him telling me that he had passed away. Would this have been a better outcome for me and my progress in my analysis? I don't necessarily think so. The flood of guilt and shame that I would have experienced knowing what he was contending with as I was giving him my usual hard time would have been very difficult for me to bear and again would have required a kind of personal engagement with me that in the midst of his grief, I doubt he could have marshalled in a way that had felt like conviction. Truly, could any of us expect that of ourselves? And yet sooner or later we will find that painful realities from our own world will move centrally into our emotional lives and inevitably impact the way we experience and respond to our patients, sometimes leading to inadvertent or ill-timed disclosures of our external circumstances. Even when carefully thought through in advance, it is impossible to know with certainty how those disclosures will land and best to proceed.

I now offer a brief vignette from my own practice. I had a young woman in ongoing psychotherapy, someone I had known since her mid-adolescence. She was a dog person and during our time together had to contend with her grief when the family dog had to be put down. And then followed the joy she experienced when a new puppy entered her life. I, too, brought a puppy into my own family and I shared this with her. We enjoyed sharing the pleasure we each took from our new canine pals. Therapeutic work continued and she would occasionally ask how my dog was getting on. When my dog was a little over 2 years old, she was hit and killed by a car over a Thanksgiving holiday when neighbors were looking after her. I knew my patient would at some point ask about her. What to do? Continue the narrative as if nothing untoward had happened, a manufactured ongoing life? I chose to tell my patient what had happened, and we shared a sad moment together. I bring this up only to point out that it had never occurred to me when I first shared that happy moment with her that I would later have to share something much more personally vulnerable. Self-disclosure is a bell that once rung can't be unrung. Miles Davis famously said about jazz improvisation, "It's not the note you play that's the wrong note – it's the note you play afterwards that makes it right or wrong". It's not the self-disclosure itself that is decisive. It's what comes next that makes all the difference.

Note

1 A version of this paper was presented at the meetings of the American Psychoanalytic Association in Boston, 2022.

References

Bollas, C. (1983). Expressive uses of the countertransference – notes to the patient from oneself. *Contemporary Psychoanalysis, 19*, 1–33.
Davies, J. M. (1994). Love in the afternoon: A relational reconsideration of desire and dread in the countertransference. *Psychoanalytic Dialogues, 4*, 153–170.
Davies, J. M. (1999). Getting cold feet, defining "safe-enough" borders: Dissociation, multiplicity, and integration in the analyst's experience. *Psychoanalytic Quarterly, 68*, 184–208.
Heimann, P. (1950). On counter-transference. *International Journal of Psychoanalysis, 31*, 81–84.
Hoffman, I. Z. (1983). The patient as interpreter of the analyst's experience. *Contemporary Psychoanalysis, 19*, 389–422.
Hoffman, I. Z. (1996). The intimate and ironic authority of the psychoanalyst's presence. *Psychoanalytic Quarterly, 65*, 102–136.
Reich, A. (1951). On counter-transference. *International Journal of Psychoanalysis, 32*, 25–31.
Slochower, J. (2017). Going too far: Relational heroines and relational excess. *Psychoanalytic Dialogues, 27*, 282–299.

Section 2

What Cannot Be Hidden

Chapters by C. Friedman, L. Emanuel, and P. Tummala-Narra

Getting comfortable with our human vulnerability has never been easy. There remain fear, shame, and confusion about disclosure, and though there has been change, we all may be vulnerable to worries when we share something that is personal.

In the previous chapters, we considered the experience of analysands who were also analysts, and how they navigated challenging disclosures. There are surprises, changes in family life, tragedies, achievements – all discoverable because milieus can and often do overlap in the dyad and in communities. We have begun to learn that, though we may want to be the gatekeepers of our lives, we live in a dynamic atmosphere where information has no boundaries anymore. Though imagination is dynamic, the transference remains hardy, reflecting individual organizational processes that are uniquely embedded, formed by history, unconscious processes, and constitution.

It is no longer a question of *whether* a patient can discover more about you than you intended, but what to do when confronted with the inevitable discoveries. The blank slate, the neutrality of the analyst in the dyad, is increasingly impacted by information, by what we cannot conceal, what we do not want to conceal. And for each dyad, and each clinician, what is uncovered, and how it is utilized in the dyad when we are tasked to consider what is obvious: skin color, ethnicity, gender, professional background. We no longer think of "if", but "when" and how. Challenging and provocative, we grapple with these changes in our authority, transference and countertransference meaning, our own visibility, and the value of sharing our human qualities. Professional and personal history has shaped each of us, integrating theory and technique, fact and fantasy, and the changing context of our work; our patients also have evolved in this changing landscape, as they bring curiosity, new ideas about what is important to them, and the unique tenor of their lives in an age where exposure and privacy have new meaning.

So too, the concept of anonymity must be considered anew. What do we mean by "blank slate"? Does the term itself denote a fundamental embodiment of a white, heteronormative, man? In recent years, we have been confronting the authority of this assumption, where difference has historically meant deviation. No longer. Exposure, or disclosure, a moment of sharing, or

DOI: 10.4324/9781003584803-6

a response to a question, a wish for privacy, or a concern about intrusion, or simply and importantly, who we are, reflect differences in each of us, the way we work, our theoretical positions, our training, or our experience. In each situation, we still consider how the unconscious is bound to the context, how experience shapes the internal world, and how the external world permeates the dyad. When who we are itself reconfigures the slate, we can reflect on our ease or discomfort, and how each dyad addresses what is known, and how this shapes the process. In the following chapters, Drs. Friedman, Emanuel, and Tummala-Narra offer their reflections on the experience of clinical work where there is no pretense. Dr. Friedman reflects on the uncanny symbolism of being a gay analyst who finds a way to open the psychic boxes of a patient; Dr. Emanuel describes how her work as a former palliative care physician has led to her psychoanalytic understanding of existential maturation, and its role in psychoanalytic treatments; and Dr. Tummala-Narra describes her experience as BIPOC therapist, and the evolution of the professional world during the course of her life as a clinician and teacher. In each case, we have an opportunity to consider how the clinician's identity becomes an integrated factor in the clinical process. Exposure, expected, embraced, visible.

4 Out of the Closet and Out of the Boxes

Reflections of a Gay Analyst on Reality and Disclosure in the Analytic Space[1]

Cary Friedman

Classical psychoanalytic technique calls upon psychoanalysts to be blank screens. Classical technique, however, was developed at a time when someone like me – an openly gay analyst – did not exist. And while subsequent relational psychoanalytic approaches acknowledged that blank screens are actually unachievable, such alternative techniques could not always account for the specific circumstances and technical dilemmas that can arise when the analyst is gay.

In January 2016, I presented my approach to patients learning about my homosexuality, either through my disclosure or through other means, to the American Psychoanalytic Association discussion group *Facing the Facts*. I began with my general stance and views about disclosure in psychoanalysis. Next, I examined issues that I see as specific to being a gay analyst, and how these issues have arisen and played out for me. Finally, I included a case presentation that illustrated how my self-disclosures helped deepen the analytic process. As someone who generally avoids writing when I can get away with it, I spoke from a prepared outline rather than reading text. Writing this chapter therefore required me to examine and more fully describe my analytic beliefs and practices nine years hence. Yet much has changed in those nine years, both in my own continuous internal development as an analyst and in our surrounding world. I have thus tried to both explicate my original presentation and describe as I go ways I might think and act differently now.

As analysts, we can seemingly control what patients learn about us both by what we disclose verbally and what they otherwise observe (i.e., our physical appearance, our office decor). I believe, though, that contemporary culture and patients today expect us to be more authentically human than in the past, and analysts feel more pressure to be "real" and not hide behind any screens. Remaining authentic while allowing room for analytic space to imagine and explore transference and unconscious fantasies can be a delicate balancing act. We are also constantly making decisions about how publicly visible to be in our lives, and what and how our patients might learn about us from outside our offices. Furthermore, since the advent of the internet, we have far less control over

DOI: 10.4324/9781003584803-7

what patients might find out from other sources than classical theorists could have imagined.

While the content of what our patients may learn about us can hugely impact their transference, I believe that equally if not more impactful is the way that the analyst handles the information. I have found patients to be acutely attuned to the subtleties of my demeanor when questions about me arise. They *feel* when I am uncomfortably guarded, uncomfortably open, or have found a more comfortable way to both acknowledge truth and find the right place to set the boundary for the moment. Modeling thoughtfulness and genuineness when navigating such moments can be profoundly helpful to our patients as they search for ways to find, understand, and accept their own identities.

General Stance and Views on Disclosure

There are many types of circumstances that arise in psychoanalytic work that call for potential disclosure, as well as many kinds of information that the analyst may consider disclosing. These include questions arising from the patient regarding concrete information about the analyst, or the analyst's inner thoughts and feelings, including their countertransference. A patient may also notice something different about their analyst and comment about it (i.e., signs of pregnancy or a wedding ring). Sometimes the analyst introduces information without a prompt from the patient – such as when the analyst's life is imposing on the treatment frame due to an illness, birth, death, or other personal situation, especially when the timing is unpredictable. And sometimes an analyst may choose for other reasons to tell the patient something – either with thoughtful intent that the disclosure will be therapeutic, or by enactment when the analyst feels pressured or anxious. Finally, patients sometimes learn things about us from outside the treatment relationship – hearing information from a third party, reading something by or about us, or looking us up online and finding disclosures we have made publicly.

There are a variety of considerations to think through about if and what to disclose. First, one tries to anticipate what the meaning might be to that particular patient of that particular piece of information at that particular time – how might it affect their transference and the analytic process? Simultaneous is the question of the patient's feelings about knowing more – is the information private? Would it feel uncomfortable, and perhaps overstimulating or anxiety-provoking to either the analyst or the patient if the information is known? On the other hand, would it feel deceptive or contrived if the analyst withholds or refuses to answer or confirm something? Might the aim of anonymity in the hopes of opening analytic exploration backfire if the patient doesn't trust the analyst because they experience them as inauthentic? Does the patient *want* to know more and see their analyst as a person with an outside life, or are they more comfortable with the anonymity? Might it help the patient to know more – such as when a patient is told the reason and time frame for a leave to help them feel reassured that the analyst will return? Is there even a clear and concrete answer to the question – such as if the patient wants to know the analyst's feelings or state of mind?

Such questions rarely have a right answer. Each occasion requires careful consideration of the context, meanings, and possible implications for each analytic dyad at that particular point in the treatment. Sometimes a choice to disclose is experienced by the patient as an unnecessary and unwanted intrusion by the analyst; sometimes a choice not to disclose constitutes collusion with the patient by ignoring the elephant in the room. Sometimes disclosing can limit analytic exploration by leaving less room for the patient's fantasies; sometimes it opens new avenues of fantasies to explore. Sometimes withholding information can signal rigid adherence to traditional analytic technique that feels contrived and unempathic. Sometimes disclosing too much information can feel unsafe and unbounded, for both the patient and the analyst. One must always try to think through – sometimes quickly and on the spot – what it might mean for the patient to ask, look, or avoid; to know or not know; to want to know or not want to know. Equally important are the patient's feelings about *how* the analyst responds to a question of disclosure, and how they might experience the analyst's comfort or discomfort with their knowing or not knowing. Thoughtful attention of all these questions is extremely helpful, and when disclosures occur more spontaneously, careful consideration needs to be given of how such interactions transpired and what unconscious forces may have led to them.

Out of the Closet: Issues Specific to Being a Gay Analyst

History and cultural context have a tremendous impact on the psychoanalytic process, a phenomenon that we were much less attuned to when I presented in 2016. Classical psychoanalytic theory largely viewed homosexuality as an illness (Friedman, 2025), and openly gay clinicians were not accepted for psychoanalytic training at most American institutes until 1991. Before then, a practicing gay analyst therefore had no choice but to be closeted to their patients and colleagues to maintain their career. Since then, several writers have discussed the pros, cons, and various complex considerations that arise around questions of disclosing the gay analyst's sexual orientation to their patients (Isay, 1991; Drescher, 1998; Phillips, 1998, 2001; Sherman, 2005). In my view, to either disclose or withhold this aspect of one's identity without careful consideration of each analytic moment risks putting the analyst's political or personal views over clinical considerations and insufficiently considering the role of countertransference in the analyst's choices. Such considerations must include how each patient and analyst have been impacted consciously and unconsciously by this history of discrimination and pathologization. Also, gay analysts may have their own degree of "outness" in their lives, and for some, information about their sexuality may feel more private.

When I presented in 2016, there was a sense that we could take for granted nonchalance about and wide acceptance of gayness. Since then, as our political environment has grown more conservative, this can no longer be assumed to be true. To complicate matters even further, since 2016, gender and sexuality are thought about much less often in discrete binary terms, so the "is the analyst straight or gay" question may call for far more complex conceptualization than it used to.

Straight analysts do not generally think about what it would mean for their patient to learn their sexual orientation in the way that gay analysts are likely to. As a gay, married man with three children, the question for me can sometimes lead to other questions about my marriage and family – if my patient knows or suspects that I am gay, and learns I have children, they may wonder *how* I became a parent. While these questions can occur for straight analysts too, patients are much more likely to make assumptions that the analyst's children were made through traditional sexual reproduction, rather than adoption, in vitro fertilization (IVF), or other means.

I came out as gay in 1985 during the third decade of my life. In 1995, I became the second openly gay person to enter psychoanalytic training at my institute, and had few models for how to address these complex questions. In 2002, two years before gay marriage became legal where I live, my now-husband and I had a commitment ceremony and subsequently married legally when that became possible in 2004. We also subsequently had three children through gestational surrogacy, a process which requires IVF. Marrying a man and parenting children together gave me less control over who knew about my sexuality, since it required identifying publicly as parents together of our kids in unexpected contexts, such as at schools or when traveling together.

Patients have come to know or wonder if I am gay through a variety of means. For some, they were aware of my sexuality on referral. Others have surmised it through their own intuition, and others learned about it from an outside source. Shortly after our first child was born, I made a spontaneous choice to identify myself publicly as gay in a particularly wide way. One day, while caring for my 2-month-old daughter at home, I received a call from a *New York Times* reporter who was interested in writing about why surrogates often like working with gay couples, and she asked if she could interview us and our surrogate. I excitedly answered yes, but then quickly thereafter panicked when I learned that the story would be on page one of the newspaper. I immediately questioned why I had agreed to this so quickly – was I overexcited about receiving the attention and not thinking about the risks of criticism I might publicly receive – for creating a gay parent-headed family, or for being so public as an analyst? But it also felt like the *right* thing to do – I was incredibly proud of my family, and it felt important to show that gay men *could* create and raise children. The article was published a few months later, and to my great relief, was very supportive of my husband and me [Bellafante, 2005]. I received only support from colleagues, and our families' fears for our safety went unrealized. What I did not anticipate, however, was how this article would impact my analytic practice. While few had noticed the article initially, many have googled me over the years since then and found it online. I have come to realize that those who have done so learned *several* distinct things about me, each of which can stir wonderings and become niduses for transference – that I am gay, I am married, I am a parent, I became a parent through artificial reproductive technology, and that I made a choice to make this information public.

I have found a range of reactions to each of these facts, but will focus here on the patient's awareness of my sexual orientation itself through whatever means they do. Most patients, when raising the topic, have been cautious and fearful of offending me, which I believe often masks the full range of their feelings. When I presented in 2016, I specifically considered how patients of different genders and sexualities have commonly reacted. For gay men, some expect that I will understand them better, and particularly appreciate that they imagine I know more about gay culture than I otherwise would. Some have described feeling particularly more comfortable talking about gay sex than they might with a straight analyst. While this may all be true, it can also lead to assumptions of shared experience that may obfuscate our differences. For gay men who are less comfortable with their sexuality, however, seeing me as comfortable with mine can feel threatening and raise anxiety. While some straight men might feel afraid that I would try to seduce them, I have found with others that they feel less pressure to display machismo, and some have fantasized that I am attracted to them and felt flattered. I have found that straight women can seemingly feel safer in the room as they imagine I am not attracted to them, while others have seemed disappointed by my presumed lack of attraction. As I consider these responses now, I realize that my patients' responses to my gayness are not necessarily so easy to categorize. Regardless of how they define their genders and sexualities, they can imagine me as attracted to them or not, feel attracted themselves to me or not, and feel comfortable or not with anything they learn about me. Modeling my comfort with any of these transferential responses is paramount to creating and fostering an analytic space.

Out of the Boxes: A Case Illustration

Ann is a 60-year-old straight, single woman who had been in analysis with me for several years at the time of my 2016 presentation. Ann came to me for evaluation of depressive symptoms, but in our first meeting she talked nonstop as she recounted her narrative of losses – a close friend, and subsequently her mother, died when she was a young child. She described how her family and community, especially her father, were so overwhelmed by their grief that Ann felt no room to experience and process her own. Upon adulthood, Ann took on the role of dutifully caring for her elderly aunt for many years despite her hatred of her, and forsook much of her own life to do so. Ann has had a successful career as an attorney, and her unique expertise in her field and charisma have made her highly sought after professionally. Her private life, however, remained inhibited and cloistered, and she has never had an intimate relationship. Ann lived in a small, dark apartment cluttered with boxes that contained the residue of her life – years of family letters, her mother's clothes, and unopened mail – that she felt afraid to open, sort through, and clear away. Ann feels quite ashamed of the clutter and rarely lets anyone into her home. Her boxes have become an important metaphor in the analysis of all the aspects of her life that she avoids examining and allowing others to see and know.

Ann quickly accepted my invitation to begin psychoanalysis, and in our first analytic meeting she related a dream that laid the groundwork for the work to come. She had gotten off a bus and arrived at a mountain of rubble. While at first the rubble was all she could see, she then noticed that behind it lay Paris, a city she'd always hoped to visit.

Ann rapidly formed a powerful but insecure attachment to me, that in time I came to understand reflected her insecure attachment to her mother. She was easily overwhelmed and overstimulated by the opportunity to imagine things she generally didn't let herself consider. Her transference included erotic elements, which particularly confused and terrified her. It also included her wishes to be taken care of by me as she feared I would abandon her prematurely as her mother did. She often talked of feeling she was "disintegrating" or "dismembering" over weekends when we didn't meet, and would use transitional phenomena – a business card she took on Fridays from my office, or a voicemail she left that she could imagine me listening to – to recompose and calm herself. I learned that she had become numb to physical pain or discomfort and rarely sought medical care, as she felt she was obviously disgusting to others and was horrified by the idea of her body being seen and touched. She was equally repulsed by looking at her own body, mind, and the contents of her boxes, yet was simultaneously desperate to see and be seen.

In my presentation in 2016, I recounted a series of disclosures through the early period of Ann's analysis and some of my reasoning at the time. As I reviewed these then, and again now in 2025, I can see how much more complex these decisions and their implications were and I might make other choices today. Accrued analytic experience and changes in our field have inevitably led to evolution in my psychoanalytic technique. I will attempt here to show my thinking at the time of these events and how I might consider them differently now.

Ann gradually learned that I am gay, married to a man, and have children, all of which has had particular meanings for her. The first such disclosure occurred one year into the analysis, when I came back from a vacation wearing a new wedding band. Ann noticed the ring immediately, saying, "That wasn't just a vacation, it was a wedding and honeymoon – right?" I asked Ann if she would like me to answer, and she said that she would. I told her that I had gotten married, and that it was to a man. Ann was outwardly excited for me, but she later told me how frightened she was – she feared that now that I was married I might abandon her, and was overstimulated by imagining me in an intimate relationship. She seemed overtly pleased to learn I was gay as it seemed familiar and safe – one of her few close friendships was with a gay man, and when they were younger she would excitedly talk with him about his sexual liberation while she hid her own lack of experience.

At the time, I thought it was appropriate to answer Ann's question directly if she wanted me to. In retrospect, however, I did not consider my disclosures about my marriage and gayness as carefully as I might now. I think that as a new analyst who had my own internal conflicts between shame and pride about my sexuality, I was overexcited by this new milestone in my life and got swept up in a moment of wanting to be seen as a proud gay man who could love and be loved. I do think, however, that Ann learning I was gay helped her feel safer in the analytic relationship, and imagining more about my marriage helped open up new areas of analytic exploration. Equally important became the spontaneity of these disclosures – I allowed some spillage from my own box of analytic "rules" which both scared and excited my patient, but gave us an abundance of more material to analyze.

Two years later, while awaiting the birth of my first child, I told Ann that I would be taking a few weeks off, longer than my usual vacations at that time. I did not disclose what my leave was for, as my supervisor and I thought that this piece of information at this point in the analysis would stir her fears of abandonment to an overwhelming degree. Ann did not ask more questions this time before or after my leave. At the time, I felt confident that I was following the principle that there was no benefit, and could be harm, from disclosing information that was not requested. In retrospect, I wonder if I had swung too hard the other way – I was still an analytic candidate and wanted my supervisor's approval, and thought it was wisest to follow traditional analytic technique. I was also at a point in my own development as an analyst where I felt more able to contain my excitement. I now wonder, however, if I was less comfortable at the time with my new identity as a parent than I had been about being gay and married.

Another two years later, I was anticipating a leave from work again as my husband and I were now expecting twins. This time, unlike the first, I could not plan my dates as carefully as before, as I expected to begin the leave when our twins were born. I consulted with a different supervisor, who advised that the unplanned start date of my leave would raise inevitable flags that something like a birth was likely, and to not tell my patient ahead of time would send a message to her that she should not talk openly about what she likely suspected anyway. Furthermore, Ann's fear of abandonment had become less intense, and I felt she could better tolerate the information this time. And, I too, had grown – I felt more comfortable with knowing how to disclose information about myself in a controlled, thoughtful way. I told Ann I was having a child. She asked me more about *how* I was having a child, and I matter-of-factly explained that we were actually having twins through gestational surrogacy. She soon asked as well if I had had a first child two years before, and I answered that I had.

In a session shortly before the birth of my twins, Ann said:

> You're going away. I have images of you and your children . . . I can't open my heart right now. I feel sealed and don't want to feel sealed. . . . There's a delicious way that I picture you and your husband – the unspeakably complex joyous chaos of three babies. I imagine lots of giggles and joy. I want to be in your family. I'm jealous in a way that I've never felt jealous before. I picture Sunday mornings, in bed, with the two year old jumping around, and the twins. Lots of feeding and diapers. I want that joyous mayhem of real life – lunchboxes, stuffy noses, measles. I'm so genuinely happy – three children who will have you as their daddy. I never let myself think of these things.

When I noted that she felt joyous *and* jealous, as well as perhaps angry, and the negative feelings might be harder to access, Ann erupted:

> Fuck you for that! You don't get it! You didn't want to hear me . . . I'm feeling scrambled and dismembered. I'm trying to tell you there's excitement next to the anger. See, you're not ready to hear something when it's different. I've been coming for three years, and I've barely been able to talk about your husband; I couldn't stand to think about him. And you – you've got it so fucking wrong. Because I want to be in your family – hear that? . . . You have no idea how hard it is to think of you having sex and babies. I feel dizzy.

As the session progressed, we noted together the "messiness and confusion" of Ann feeling so much all at once. In addition to joy and jealousy, Ann described her love of and attachment to me, as well as "fury" and terror about my upcoming leave. The next day, Ann apologized for her explosion of emotions, and noted how she felt "conflicted" and "scrambled with jealousy and anger". She then explained:

> When I was thinking about your family, I just wanted you to let me have that. Because otherwise, I feel overstimulated and scared. The fact that you didn't with 200% accept it, leads me to feeling dismembered. I can describe the reason. When I need to sit up and see you, connect with your eyes – it helps me to feel calmer – you know me. When you say you get it and hear it, it's like you're connecting to me, and when you say that you don't get it, I feel dismembered. When I think of Susan's [her friend] daughters, of your two-year-old, or a baby on the train crying, I think – they're babies and can't say what's wrong or where the pain is! You try giving them a nap, or a bottle, or change them, you just keep trying. They can't tell you what's wrong but they're waiting. I used

> to wonder – at what point would Susan just throw the baby away? Then the parent figures it out – this kind of squeal means this, that means that, etc. it's not the baby's job to say "Dad – I need this!" But when do parents say, "three shots and you're gone?"

In these sessions, Ann's wide range of reactions to my disclosures about my life shows how this knowledge deepened rather than inhibited the analytic process. Ann describes vividly, and longingly, her fantasy of the "joyous mayhem" of my upcoming family life. She imagines me as deeply immersed and happy. I believe that Ann *was* genuinely happy for me. But she also felt jealous that I will have a parenting experience that she does not, jealous of my husband for having me romantically, jealous of my children for having me care for them in ways I won't for her, and overstimulated by all these swirling internal conflicts. It seemed to me that Ann was trying to manage these conflicts by keeping her competing emotions apart in metaphorical intra-psychic boxes. She was frightened of experiencing the greater complexity of her affective responses, and she felt angry when I noted her apparent disavowal. She felt terrified of her own rage and tried to pull it back. Her associations then showed her desperate longing to be understood, even if she could not articulate her needs. They also showed the depth of her fear of abandonment if she does not contain herself – she wondered if she would become so difficult that, like Susan's child or mine, we would say "three shots and you're gone?" Furthermore, Ann's fantasy of my family life seemed itself to be another transitional phenomenon that contained her and helped stave off her fears of dismemberment.

Over the next several years, Ann slowly, gradually, and sometimes in fits and starts became less fearful and better integrated. Fears of abandonment and urges to contain and hide remained constant themes, but with gradually less intensity, and she stopped taking cards from my office and calling on weekends. Ann continued to talk intermittently about my family – remembering my kids' ages and imagining specifics of their developmental progression with uncanny accuracy. She imagined that there were disagreements in our household, but that we would lovingly talk them through, and I would *never* say "three shots and your gone" to my husband or children. She could better tolerate disagreements with me, and she became more open to seeking medical help when needed, including allowing a necessary surgical procedure. While any slight reference to the possibility of terminating treatment at some point led to panic and flooded her, she came to tolerate in time the possibility of decreasing our meeting frequency from four times weekly. And shortly before I presented in 2016, Ann noticed a sign for an available apartment that was both larger and more up to date than her own. She took a huge leap out of her familiar lair and moved.

Still, many boxes remained in the old apartment that she hadn't yet given up – while she now occupied her new home, she had stalled on moving her belongings. Her boxes were old and falling apart, so Ann bought large trash bags to enclose them. When I asked where they actually were at that point, Ann gave a long, vague and uninterruptible description that felt guarded to me – as if she didn't want me to try to open anything, concretely or emotionally. She then said,

> Where did the boxes go? I had planned to empty them all before moving, and maybe I could have if I had used our time to think about this with you. So after my trip, I started the process of just bringing them to the new apartment. I covered the couch with a sheet and rolled up the rug. The only place for the boxes in bags was smack in the center. The other thirty will go in storage. So my goal, and I think it's very feasible, and I'm motivated because I want the pictures to go up, is to go through them this week. I'm not concerned.

When Ann finally paused, I thought about how often over the years Ann has said she will do something promptly that she never gets to, and I sensed that at that moment she could tolerate my challenge. I said, "I am. It's not been that simple for you to just clear out the boxes when you say you will. The boxes have been a useful metaphor for us about how you keep things closed up and covered, and opening them has many meanings, and stirs many feelings that are hard to process. So it sounds now like you may be filling and covering your new apartment like the old one". Ann responded, "Right now I feel – this is a moment that would have made me very defensive in the past. Yes – I'm always not doing things. When I got movers, I thought it would be much easier. I love this new building; if I didn't have the lure of the new apartment, I don't know if I'd get to the boxes". I noted that finding the apartment itself spoke to figuratively opening a box, but that "the fact that boxes are actually still there speaks to the ways you feel ready to open many things and ways you don't – you wrestle back and forth". Ann said, "I realize the comfort of being in the presence of the boxes . . . I know I've been in a fort for thirty years. When I opened one box, I found a notice of my phone being disconnected, a letter from my mother, and a letter to you. The boxes became radioactive, as if I couldn't touch them. But then they became less radioactive". I suggested that it might be useful for us to look at things from the boxes together, as I wondered what meanings the objects within might have. She said, "I understand that the objects connect me to my heritage. I have pictures of my mother, and pieces of my family's crystal, pieces only I can own, *so I know who I am*". I said, "It makes me think of the meanings of objects here between us, how they can make you feel together and whole". Ann said, "Yes. The cards from my mother tell me where I come from". I said, "Your identity is tied to these objects; some are comfortable and some are not. I think we have more to do – there's so much more in the boxes". Ann replied, "Absolutely".

This session shows the intricacies of the psychic functions that objects carry for Ann. She holds her literal boxes ambivalently – she both wants and doesn't want to have them, open them, gaze inside them, connect with their contents, and understand their meanings. When she does allow us to consider their contents, it is clear that they contain a plethora of meanings – they connect her to her mother, her past, and her heritage. They also contain a letter to me – perhaps one that was written in an attempt to connect to me, but instead got tucked away and hidden. Ann also describes how these objects, and both what and who they represent, help her feel grounded, whole, and with a stronger sense of identity. While her continued ambivalence is evident, her progress is as well. She is markedly more tolerant of both interpretations from me and new possibilities in her outside life.

This session, ten years following the previous ones I described, contains no direct references to Ann's knowledge about my sexuality and family, or the way she learned about them. I believe, however, that the impact of my disclosures is operative here in displacement – if I could comfortably open my closet, Ann could open her boxes. I think that Ann's transference experience of me as someone sufficiently unimpeded by shame and inhibition to feel comfortable in my identity, as demonstrated by how I have handled self-disclosures over time, set a model for how Ann can face her own shame and inhibitions. This model powerfully reverberates in Ann's unconscious and continues to help her open more boxes, be they cardboard or conceptual.

Conclusion

Psychoanalytic technique necessarily changes over time as factors in our outside world and analytic understanding of the mind evolve, and consideration of self-disclosure of the analyst's sexual orientation has required new questions to be tackled that had not been in the past. In my experience as a gay psychoanalyst, my sexuality has been the most common question regarding self-disclosure that I have faced. I aim to approach it as I do any other potential disclosure or known information about me – carefully and thoughtfully, with full attention to the possible implications, benefits, and disadvantages of my responses. I prioritize the importance of both clear boundaries and authenticity, and allow for how respecting both can lead to "imperfect" technique. Experience, however, has helped me to embrace imperfection in psychoanalytic work. Allowing space for stumbles and play, and working to understand their unconscious meanings, can lead to valuable growth, as I believe has been evident with Ann. We all have closets and boxes, and the better we as analysts can navigate the complexities of our own, the better we can help our patients do so.

Note

1 A version of this paper was presented at the 2016 National meeting of the American Psychoanalytic Association in New York City.

References

Bellafante, G. (2005, May 27). Surrogate mothers' new niche: Bearing babies for gay couples. *New York Times*. Retrieved from http://nytimes.com/2005/05/27/us/surrogate-mothers-new-niche-bearing-babies-for-gay-couples.html.

Drescher, J. (1998). *Psychoanalytic therapy & the gay man*. Hillsdale, NJ/London: The Analytic Press.

Friedman, C. (2025). A gay old time: Evolving psychoanalytic paradigms of (homo) sexuality. [in press, *Psychoanalytic Inquiry*].

Isay, R. (1991). The homosexual analyst: Clinical considerations. *Psychoanalytic Study of the Child*, *46*, 199–216.

Phillips, S. H. (1998). A new analytic dyad: Homosexual analyst, heterosexual patient. *Journal of the American Psychoanalytic Association*, *46*, 1195–1219.

Phillips, S. H. (2001). The overstimulation of everyday life: 1. New aspects of male homosexuality. *Journal of the American Psychoanalytic Association*, *49*, 1235–1267.

Sherman, E. (2005). *Notes from the margins: The gay analyst's subjectivity in the treatment setting*. Hillsdale, NJ/London: The Analytic Press.

5 Existential Maturation

As a Guide to Aging- and Illness-Related Self-Disclosure Practices

Linda Emanuel

Introduction

The following sets out the way in which I guide my decisions about aging- and illness-related self-disclosure. Having come to the practice of psychoanalysis after a career in palliative medicine, my assumptions about if and how to self-disclose with patients were guided by awareness of how our mortal state impacts people and our relationships with those who depend on us. A core notion, existential maturation, developed initially from within palliative medicine but explicated from within psychoanalysis, offered what I found to be a reliable compass for many aspects of the analyst-analysand interaction (Emanuel et al., 2017; Emanuel, 2023). Self-disclosure about aging- and illness-related self-disclosure was one such aspect.

What Is Existential Maturation?

Palliative medicine was pioneered by Cicely Saunders and became a specialty in medicine on the experience that it is possible to die well, bringing quality experiences to both the dying and the bereaved (Clark, 2018). This contrasts with the alternative route, more often presumed as inevitable; that of dying with profound suffering that afflicts both the dying and the bereaved. This quality of dying seemed to be determined by a person's, family's, or community's existential maturation. At an individual level, existential maturation is a life-long process, the defining goal of which is a mature relationship to the reality of mortality. It designates a developmental journey that often results in prioritized relational living. It is developed through myriad manageable engagements with mortality – perhaps the death of a pet or a close-call vehicular accident accompanied by caring support. It appears to be fostered by healthy attachment or containing relationships. It is impeded by traumatic experiences of death – perhaps in combat or when an essential person in one's life is lost and support is inadequate. States of advanced existential maturation bring delight in life alongside equanimity about its regretted but accepted end. People oscillate back and forth in their states of existential maturation. This is especially so after a salient mortality reminder such as a new illness

DOI: 10.4324/9781003584803-8

diagnosis, and the degree of oscillation lessens as the new reality is metabolized (Jackson & Emanuel, 2024).

My entry into psychoanalysis was partly to help understand how the reality of mortality gets metabolized and to trace the nature of this developmental process. It turned out that existential maturation was also a widely relevant aspect of the mind and a helpful concept in many matters – including as a guide for me in thinking through things like how to handle self-disclosure.

Existential Maturation as My Guide to Self-Disclosure

My introduction to self-disclosure in the analytic relationship was a surprise. Looking back, I think the clash of different vantage points opened up space that allowed existential maturation to emerge as my guide. The following anonymized story set the stage: a weekly case conference, a group of trainees, and the presentation of a clinical encounter to an experienced clinician:

We all saw the teacher's face fall. Still loosely holding notes of her first encounter with her control case, my peer was taken aback by the detailed questions our teacher asked about something she'd written *no* notes on: how she introduced herself. He in turn was taken aback by her answers. The patient had asked about her background, and she candidly shared her status as an analytic candidate, and then, as part of what she felt was fair and full disclosure, she added licensure, training, and additional background that she thought was relevant and reassuring. The class wanted to know what was wrong with that. The answer: with her disclosure, she'd reinforced an idealizing transference and lost the opportunity to explore what it meant to the patient that she was in training. Bravely I thought, my peer admitted that yes, she too needed reassurance of her adequacy to take on this work.

After decades of abiding by the role-dictated behaviors in my first career in medicine, I was blindly familiar with the way these norms selectively encouraged or discouraged transferences and counter-transferences. The physician was to be idealized – trustworthy and invincible against illness and death. The patient was to elicit the clinician's desire to administer care, buoyed by the role. Dress codes and identification badges and trained practices regarding greetings and bodily communications facilitated the processes (Stoeckle, 1987). Medical interventions were material, and the therapeutic relationship was a context, not an intervention in and of its own nature.

More decades later, I am impressed by the care with which we psychoanalysts tend to transference, our instrument of perception and medium of transformation. But I am less impressed by the need to protect it with rigid norms. Transference finds its way to the fore remarkably well if the analyst is paying attention. And often it does so better in the absence of technique-oriented manipulations. Transference withers, perhaps responding to its impersonal nature, in the face of prescribed transactions more than in the face of genuine, even if aberrant, communications.

At the same time, our teacher was also correct: self-disclosure can also interfere with the frame. Along with other tangible features such as schedule, payment, and physical setting, expectations about what is knowable about the analyst and what is not, help to maintain the frame (Gill, 1983). So, if the analyst offers or obliges by offering requested self-disclosures, the frame can become unreliable. Or, conversely, if the analyst withholds relevant information about themselves, the frame can become sterile or be betrayed (Levenson, 1996).

In short, self-disclosure has an undeniable influence on the analytic dyad's ability to access useable transference and countertransference, and my peer's rooky error was real. Nonetheless, as the case presentation progressed, we could see (and our teacher pointed it out too) that my peer's control case patient went forward with well-used idealization as well as other transference-based work. So, I had reason to reflect on which norms of self-disclosure I wanted to retain from medicine in my psychoanalytic practice.

Since most of my medical days were spent in geriatric and palliative medicine, I had plenty of material regarding aging and dying to consider with regard to self-disclosure. I also had my "north star concept" of existential maturation. Rules-based guidance could only go so far, as our teacher also affirmed, in relationships tailored for engaging the dynamic mind. Furthermore, with psychoanalysis being my second career, I was no spring chicken, and some personal matters were likely to and did become relevant. These are the reflections and experiences I share below. In the spirit of optimal self-disclosure, I use real examples from my own experience.

What Illnesses to Disclose

Capacity Limiting Conditions

The medical world I came from was not perfect at keeping ill and incapacitated clinicians from practice, but it had a more robust system than we do in many psychoanalytic settings. With sparse if any routine recertification requirements and with the limitations of peer review and institutional monitoring imposed by the private nature of our practice, psychoanalysts have to gauge when our own capacity is limiting (American Board of Psychoanalysis).

At 71 years old my word recall and my memory of scheduling items are not what it was when I was 50. It is still good enough, but I have lapses. Initially, I was embarrassed by its diminishment, worried it would be damaging and would undermine patient's confidence in me. But it was real, so I made a choice to make easy mention of the phenomena. Comments such as "did we say 4 or 5p for the Tuesday session?" or articulating word finding difficulties with a preamble such as "hold on, my aging mind is searching for the word . . . ah yes, . . ." made small open declarations that am aware of and will take responsibility for my fallibility. My hope is that this practice sets expectations for if and when more serious limits to my capacity emerge; that I will disclose whatever the issue is and not leave my patients to discover it through its unmanaged adverse consequences. To the best of my awareness this practice makes the frame more, not less solid and has not interfered with useability of transferences.

Furthermore, it offers the patient an experience of the analyst's existential maturation. This can be an essential opportunity for idealization, internalization, and development of the capacity in patients themselves. Realizing that became, for me, a step along my growing confidence in the ability of this concept of existential maturation to be my guide.

Schedule/Frame Impinging Conditions

Some self-disclosure is prompted by practical impingements on the schedule. When I broke my leg a short answer (an accident while playing with my rather large dog) to questions of how come was usually appropriate. It generated, for some, new material about the dangers of big dogs, especially for the elderly, or for others the meaning of canine love. All were "grist for the mill" and went some way toward compensating for lost analytic time while I was away.

When a new cardiac condition – that turned out to be benign – needed a several week schedule-interrupting work-up, I shared the reality with patients in different ways. For some patients, I chose not to communicate about it at all (saying only "I need to reschedule this time") but would have if they had asked or if it had not been benign. For other patients it generated concern that I might retire and even if the analysis were to complete the possibility of return would been taken away. For others, it became an opportunity to consider their disappointment that I was mortal. This became an interpretation opportunity for me, which I made use of selectively but often, to engage their own death anxieties.

The more my experience as an analyst built, the more I felt, in keeping with some aspects of existential analysis, that no analysis was complete without addressing a person's relationship to mortality (Yalom, 1980). So self-disclosures about illness became important components of the work.

In all these self-disclosure examples, the transference shifted but was used. One person might find it an opening to acknowledge their need for an unending internal object. For another it might become a chance to engage with optimal frustration the permanence of termination. To my understanding, these were welcome "optimal distance" exposures to mortality that fostered my patients' existential maturation.

For the patients with whom I did not share my condition, it had seemed too likely that it would prompt an unhelpful repetition or a trauma. While those could have been handled, timing is important. As long as the condition was benign, and I felt this would have been unfortunate timing for those patients, non-disclosure seemed appropriate. This is a line of reasoning to use with care, however. It is all too easy for the analyst who is caught up in their own denial to project their own need for protection onto the patient and never disclose.

Duration Limiting Conditions

Expected limitations on a treatment's duration are worth revealing, in my opinion. Analysts who know they will retire at a set time or analysts with a chronic condition that is behind a decision to stop work after a while rarely do their patients a favor by withholding that information. A recent seminar on the topic described an analyst who told her patients that she will retire in two years. I admire that. Considerable appreciation was expressed by seminar participants who noted the benefits to patients who then have the time to discover what that stirs in them and to process it with adequate time. This practice has great potential to entirely preempt the traumatic effects to the patient of finding one's analyst suddenly hospitalized or deceased without warning. In short, if disclosure offers the patient a building of their existential maturation, it's probably the right thing to do.

Of note, all of these rules of thumb about existential maturation moments for the patient depend on the analyst having the capacity to nurture it. That means the analyst has to have their own ongoing sufficient existential maturation.

Emergency Changes

Some years ago, a family medical emergency out of state meant that I made an abrupt move that would take me away from my in-person practice. Most of my practice continued by video. I thought initially it would be for a month or so, but it turned out to be a year and at the end of that year the COVID pandemic began. For some patients deeply engaged in tender work it was painfully disruptive. A candid self-disclosure about the reasons why I moved and why I no longer planned to return seemed the least I could offer and far less damaging than the alternative of withholding the information. It was a situation with a newborn grandchild that had sent me off in such haste; it had a happy outcome but took a few years before that became so.

How the event and the disclosed information were followed with its processing mattered a great deal. For most analysands deep in their work, such a sudden departure would be traumatic. Strong work to find and process its meaning to them was essential. A solid basis in the reality of why it happened was helpful to them and to me as well. This was a time when I had and made good use of, but needed and should have asked for more, support from my peers, consultants, and my own analyst. Some new trauma did result to my patients; but I do not think that withholding self-disclosure would have helped. Rather it would have made it worse. I also think that both my own and most or all of the patients' existential maturation grew and that, as hard as it was, self-disclosure was an important or even essential part of the process.

Professional Wills

Professional wills become a kind of self-disclosure for older analysts, and indeed for all analysts. At the time my cardiac condition came up, some people asked what would happen if I died suddenly. I was able to remind them about my professional will. Having told them about it at the beginning of treatment, when I also required a consent for treatment form and set the payment frame, it became a reminder rather than a new matter. Having and acknowledging and discussing the relevant content of a professional will are an occasion when the analyst's existential maturity is on display. What is being disclosed is my acceptance that I am mortal and my effort to make that a non-traumatizing reality for people around me. In my experience, patients have found it reassuring.

Misuses of Non-Disclosure

Analyst's Self-Protection

There's an adage in my erstwhile field of palliative medicine that by the time you need a health care proxy designation it's too late to arrange for one. A health care proxy is a person who makes decisions for you if you are no longer competent to make your own. A strong movement to get people to make those designations while in normal health when it seemed irrelevant was needed to avoid the common situation of a person becoming too ill to still have the competence to legally hand over decision-making to their chosen proxy. If that chosen person was not the legal next of kin, an already difficult situation often became much more so. It takes either enforced norms of practice or a good deal of existential maturation including a sense of responsibility for loved ones' care to make plans ahead of time for one's own most vulnerable times. Many people put it off or avoid it entirely.

A similar situation arises in psychoanalytic practices when the analyst is in declining health, perhaps including mental capacity, and is in sufficient denial that arrangements are not made. Anecdotally, a great many analysts fail to retire in a timely manner and patients have to deal with a dawning realization that their analyst is not "with it". Or they have to wait during a hospitalization that was misrepresented as minor for their analyst to return, but the analyst never comes back. These situations are potentially enormously damaging to the patient (Goldberg, 2023). The patient may feel tricked and abandoned and it may be hard to hold onto the gains of the treatment prior to its untimely end. In general, not only is there an interruption in treatment that they were unprepared for, the patient must deal with the obvious reality that the analyst could have but did not prepare for such an event with a modest amount of requisite self-disclosure.

The only build to a patient's existential maturation that might occur from failure to have appropriately disclosed in this kind of situation is a counterphobic one.

Patient Exploitation/Inconsideration

Dutiful self-disclosure of age-related or illness-related issues may serve to preempt or minimize the exploitations that can happen without the analyst's awareness. Consider a patient of an analyst with early but progressing dementia. The patient may be startled one day to find the analyst making inappropriate comments or touching in inappropriate ways or not arriving on time or expecting the patient to serve in some other role, perhaps as an employee or a family member. Had the analyst made a habit of openly owning small cognitive losses or sharing the diagnosis of early dementia, the patient would have had a better chance to end the work in a timely fashion or at least understand the odd behaviors as something resulting from the analyst's mental decline. Quite a few analysts have worked with patients who experienced such things and who, fortunately, went on to another analysis to help unpack the damage done (Galatzer-Levy, 2004). In these subsequent treatments that eventually ensued, analysts have found that the patient was at that time too deep in a transferential relationship with the former analyst to experience it as anything that was a limitation of the analyst. Rather they experienced it as something like an injuring intent to diminish or exploit or violate their boundaries.

Again, the only build to a patient's existential maturation from this kind of failure to disclose is a counterphobic one.

Varied Norms by School of Thought

Disclosures of the Mind

Needs regarding self-disclosure are significantly different depending on the analyst's practice orientation. A Freudian intervention aims to discover the patient's mind (Kernberg, 2016). A Winnicottian approach entails playfulness, which can be quite revealing of the analyst (Winnicott, 1971). A Kohutian intervention entails vicarious introspection or empathy from the analyst as the instrument of discovery and cure (Kohut, 1984). A Bionian intervention entails co-creation between the patient's emerging and the analyst's containing minds (Bion, 1970). Sufficient non-disclosure remains necessary in all approaches to maintain the frame and prevent boundary crossing. But it can be quite difficult to learn how to do that in later, more collaborative psychoanalytic approaches that also work with much more injured patients than Freud's.

Consider a patient with a dead mother complex and a powerful need to be seen and understood by the therapist (Green, 1980). The analyst must work through their own related injuries in order to see and appreciate in an experience-near fashion the patient's struggle. The issues in this kind of situation are with psychic deadness rather than physical mortality. However, existential maturation with regard to physical mortality is mediated through the experience of psychic deadness, in my opinion (Emanuel, et al, in press). So here too, I find that existential maturation offers a compass.

Psychic deadness and its proximity to murderous rage and a felt imperative to or hopelessness about being able to connect deeply with another make it easy to imagine a patient in such a difficult psychic place seeking more knowledge of the analyst's mind. This may become a matter of self-disclosure for the analyst. For instance, a patient may demand that the analyst "own their own defenses" or share their own parallel experiences.

In such situations, I have had to rely on estimating the patient's own existential maturation to "accurately intuit" what to share and what to withhold. Often it is appropriate to disclose that there is enough parallel experience that the analyst can see and feel what is true for the patient without disclosing specifics. For example, the analyst may say: "I think I know something of how that must feel; in such a situation I find that. . . . Perhaps you feel some of that too?" The guiding goal is to allow that the analyst too works with experiences that come from feeling deadened or experiencing mortality as an inner deadness, but without breaking the frame. For the patient, appreciating what comes from the analyst's observed or personal experience of metabolizing psychic deadness can allow the twinning and identification that becomes a source of vital growth.

How to Gauge Efficacy of Non-Disclosure/Self-Disclosure

Patient Flourishes, Patient Terminates

The imperative to create therapeutic, analytic love, complete with the fields of transference in which we work, yet in a manner that reliably avoids boundary transgressions, has given rise to a number of rules. Not the least of these rules are limitations on self-disclosure. So, in urging the case for meaningful self-disclosure when it comes to analyst age-related limits or illness, as I do here, it is important to be careful. I have suggested that the analyst can be guided by their own experience-based understanding of existential maturation. And the counterpart guiding theme is this: the patient's existential maturation is also a barometer. If the patient is flourishing and terminates with a greater sense of vitality with acceptance of their own and their loved ones' finitude, that can be a pretty good gauge that whatever disclosure was done or not done, it pretty much worked.

Much of my practice is characterized by patients who are grappling with defining illnesses either in themselves or in a loved one. Engaging existential matters is a core part of what we do. To be able to talk about death and loss and engage existential suffering on a daily basis, I draw greatly on the discovery of most every palliative care clinician. That is, that doing so is not pathologically morbid but a process than engages life and love more than a sanitized, death-denying analytic process and promotes forward-moving development.

Sometimes it takes a while for a death-aversive person to experience – and even longer for them to trust the experience – of life affirmation that comes from processing death and loss. It can take months or years, sometimes many years, for a person to develop their own capacity and ways to do this with people in their lives outside of analysis. Since, as I see it, an analysis is not complete until the analysand is well-enough accepting of their and their essential others' mortality, it is worth working on until that point.

Another reality, already alluded to, is that all this engagement fosters my development in that domain as well, and it feeds my vitality and my death acceptance as well. When I disclose my aging- and illness-related issues, my existential maturation is disclosed as well. The analysand gets to identify with that aspect of me, and to make it their own, safely internalized for their own use with themselves and the people they connect with. So, it is imperative that my own existential maturation be good enough and always active and in process, and one way of checking in on how my patients are doing is checking the kind of existential maturation I find in my countertransference with that patient.

Why Does Existential Maturation Guide Self-Disclosure in Matters of Aging and Illness?

While existential maturation was a concept developed to understand how come some people die with a sense of enviable peace and transmission of love that carries their loved ones forward in bereavement, it turned out to be a concept with relevance to the full life-cycle experience. To consider how it is relevant for self-disclosure, here is a short re-rendition of its process.

Existential maturation is a process that starts with a confrontation between the will to live – in connection with an essential other – and the fact of death. Klein describes in the way in which toggling between the paranoid-schizoid position (reasonably understood by Klein as the death drive) and the depressive position becomes the engine for development. The process by which a person develops a manageable acceptance of and way of living well while knowing the reality of death is similar to that described by Bion. Bion described how a child uses their parent-figure's alpha function to metabolize the raw realities of life that Bion called beta elements. So too, existential maturation appears to make experiences of psychic or actual death manageable with containing relationships and the structures that come from repeated such interactions. This drives a mode of living that is realistically grounded in the limits to our vital capacities for enlivening relationship. Unmanageable experiences of death can be traumatizing or deadening. But if it goes well, as a core part of our mechanism for developing a life of meaning among others, and as a psychological process with known ways to go wrong, existential maturation offers the analyst a natural guide to healthy process in many psychological matters. Why does this include self-disclosure in matters of aging and illness?

The analyst engages the patient in a process of discovery and development, using the mind of the analyst as a Kleinian and Bionian parent figure to hold and co-create the parts of the analysand that need it. The risk of self-disclosure is that it distorts the process by bringing in too much of the analyst. Then the analysand does not find the undistorted self in the co-creation. This risk has unique features when regarding aging and illness that directly impact the central process of existential maturation, namely managing the fact of and implications of being finite in capacity and duration. If the analyst brings a dishonest, inauthentic, distorted, or exploitative version of their own process to the co-creations of the analytic process, the patient's process will also be impaired.

On the reverse side, the desirable process of taking in and making vital use of known and acknowledged limitations allows for a healthy co-creative process with the patient. To do this, the analyst must be comfortable enough with their own limitations and mortality to acknowledge it appropriately.

In short, existential maturation offers a guide to self-disclosure regarding aging- and illness-related matters because doing so is part and parcel of the analytic process.

Concrete and Less Concrete Actions

The practical upshot is simple enough and should be part of psychoanalysts' practice ethics. When the psychoanalyst's illness impacts the treatment – for instance, its schedule, the analyst's ability to bring their analytic mind, or the treatment's expected duration – ego-syntonic (for the patient, that is) disclosure is indicated. When starting treatment, at a time when matters like payment and confidentiality are being discussed and consent for treatment forms are being signed, the analysand should know that the analyst has a professional will that covers what happens to any information about them and who would contact them in the event of death.

Less concretely, but importantly, the analyst must know and be engaged with their own existential maturation. Society allows that the fear of death and the avoidance of the topic are normal and acceptable coping. Although Freud treated matters of mortality in his works and arguably all major analytic thinkers since then have too, the training and practice of psychoanalysis do not include proportionate attention to mortality matters. So many analysts fall into the same bind their analysands do of having rudimentarily and fearful relationships with their own mortality. Wherever each analyst is, with regard to their own existential mortality, it is important to be engaged with the process, contemplating and engaging with and discussing life-and-death matters with essential others and colleagues in all the training and life-long learning settings available to us. An existentially maturing analyst will engage the existential maturation of the analysand. Self-disclosure of aging- and illness-related matters will be part of both. When the analysand has achieved good-enough existential maturation and is ready to terminate, the analyst will know that she or he has done a good enough job with self-disclosure.

References

American Board of Psychoanalysis. American Board of Psychoanalysis – Home Further Instructions in Preparing a Professional Will APsA-Code-of-Ethics.pdf

Bion, W. R. (1970). Container and contained: Attention and interpretation: A scientific approach to insight. *Psycho-Analysis and Groups, 2*, 72–82.

Clark, D. (2018). *Cicely saunders: A life and legacy*. Oxford University Press. ISBN: 0190637935.

Emanuel, L. (2023). Existential maturation: A dynamic psychophysiology model. *Journal of Palliative Medicine, 26*(12), 1604–1609.

Emanuel, L., Galatzer-Levy, R., & Lebovitz, P. (In Press). The existential maturation project – death matters: A psychoanalytic perspective. *Psychoanalytic Inquiry*.

Emanuel, L., Reddy, N., Hauser, J., & Sonnenfeld, S. (2017). And yet it was a blessing: The case for existential maturity. *Journal of Palliative Medicine, 20*(4), 318–327.

Galatzer-Levy, R. M. (2004). The death of an analyst: Patients whose previous analyst died while they were in treatment. *Journal of the American Psychoanalytic Association, 52*, 999–1024.

Gill, M. M. (1983). The interpersonal paradigm and the degree of the therapist's involvement. *Contemporary Psychoanalysis, 19*, 200–237.

Goldberg, S. (2023). Fresh sufferings: Psychoanalysis in the retirement phase. Sarah Goldberg dissertation by ICSW – Issuu.

Green, A. (1980). *The dead mother in on private madness*. Karnac Books.

Jackson, V., & Emanuel, L. (2024). Navigating and communicating about serious illness and end of life. *New England Journal of Medicine, 390*, 63–69. https://doi.org/10.1056/NEJMcp2304436

Kernberg, O. F. (2016, Sep 22). The four basic components of psychoanalytic technique and derived psychoanalytic psychotherapies. *World Psychiatry, 15*(3), 287–288. https://doi.org/10.1002/wps.20368

Kohut, H. (1984). *How does analysis cure?* University of Chicago Press.

Levenson, E. A. (1996). Aspects of self-revelation and self-disclosure. *Contemporary Psychoanalysis, 32*, 237–248.

Stoeckle, J. (Ed.) (1987). *Encounters between patients and doctors: An anthology*. Cambridge, MA & London, England: The MIT Press.

Winnicott, D. W. (1971). *Playing and reality*. Routledge 2005.

Yalom, I. (1980). *Existential psychotherapy*. Basic Books.

6 Dilemmas of Self-Disclosure

The Hypervisibility and Invisibility of Race and Culture

Pratyusha Tummala-Narra

Amidst presenting a case in a psychodynamic group supervision early in my career, I was interrupted by the supervisor, who suddenly exclaimed that she admired my skin. Feeling stunned, I said, "thank you", and continued to present the case material to the group. No one in the all-White supervision group spoke to me about the supervisor's comments. I was alone with my heightened sense of being brown. I wondered about the supervisor's fascination and her discomfort with my skin color so much so that she felt she had to interrupt a case presentation that contained no reference to race or skin color other than my brief mention of the patient's race and ethnicity. This incident is reminiscent of many others throughout my career when supervisors, colleagues, and patients have reacted to my skin color and my Asian Indian ethnicity in both explicit and subtle ways.

In my training in the 1990s, I was taught that the therapist or analyst should not disclose personal information to the patient as this would disrupt the therapeutic frame and neutrality, essential to transference. Yet, I understood that my skin color, race, and ethnicity mark a "colored screen", a concept developed by Comas-Díaz and Jacobsen (1991), referring to a patient's intensified projections in response to a therapist's physical features. My race and culture have always been in the foreground of how people have perceived me in the United States. Therefore, my brown skin color and ethnicity cannot be hidden in the context of psychotherapy. Rather, my phenotype becomes a screen for a range of different projections, in contrast to a "blank slate". Yet, perceptions of my brown skin tone and Indian heritage shape complex transferential responses and relational connections and disconnections. Notably, race is typically more visible, whereas cultural, religious, and political values and beliefs are less visible to patients. As such, each of these aspects of identity or social location has different implications for the therapist's self-disclosure. The focus of this chapter is on dilemmas that arise regarding self-disclosure of race and culture in the therapeutic dyad. Specifically, I highlight how fantasies of race and ethnicity are juxtaposed against felt subjectivities of the therapist and patient, how race and culture are often tied with past and current traumas that present themselves in the therapeutic relationship, and how self-disclosure regarding race and culture has the potential to facilitate the recognition of sociocultural experiences,

DOI: 10.4324/9781003584803-9

but also to disrupt the patient's free association and the nature of the connection with the therapist.

Theoretical Questions Concerning Self-Disclosure

As the aim of this chapter is not to provide an extensive review of psychoanalytic literature concerning self-disclosure, I briefly highlight some concepts which are especially useful in considering self-disclosure regarding race and culture. Theoretical questions about therapist self-disclosure have been raised throughout the history of psychoanalysis. In a historical overview of this topic, Richards (2018) described theoretical orthodoxy and rigidity in American psychoanalysis following World War II, and how by the 1960s and 70s, non-self-disclosure or the blank screen was an important guiding principle. Richards (2018, p. 153) noted, "We cannot make our decision on principle, only on the particulars". Furthermore, he made a distinction between inadvertent self-disclosure (e.g., how we appear or speak) and deliberate self-disclosure (e.g., our beliefs, personal life experiences, our feelings about the patient).

Relatedly, Frankel (2018) detailed Balint's (1968) distinction between benign and malignant regression, relevant to the analyst's self-disclosure. Benign regression reflects a patient's need for recognition by the analyst that facilitates introspection and discovery of unconscious material, whereas malignant regression reflects a type of idealization of the analyst in which the patient "looks to the analyst to solve his inner problems", limiting the patient's ability to work through conflict and trauma (Frankel, 2018, p. 357). Frankel (2018), elaborating on the distinction between these two types of regression, notes how the analyst's self-disclosure carries unique implications for each patient. In other words, self-disclosure can be essential to a basic sense of safety and trust but it also holds the potential for collusion in either avoiding painful and conflictual material or repeating traumatic experiences. The openness to therapist self-disclosure as beneficial to the patient was expanded through intersubjective and relational perspectives (Mitchell, 1988; Stolorow, 1988). While some re-traumatization may be inevitable as therapeutic work requires both risk and safety (Bromberg, 2010; West, 2017), the therapist's warmth and responsiveness are critical for the relationship, particularly when the patient has suffered traumatic experiences (West, 2017).

Despite these developments, race and culture have largely been excluded from theory concerning self-disclosure. Psychoanalytic theory concerning self-disclosure has largely neglected race and culture, in part because sociocultural traumas, such as racism, have not been conceptualized as forms of psychic trauma (Bromberg, 2010). Systematically, there has been an absence of the subjectivity of racial minority therapists and patients, which includes sociocultural traumas. More recently, racial minority and White analysts and psychoanalytic therapists have written about their experiences of race, skin color, gender, immigration, culture, language, religion, social class, disability, and intersectionality, raising awareness of the impacts of collective sociocultural traumas on theoretical conceptualizations and therapeutic work (Akhtar, 2014; Leary, 1997; Holmes, 2012; Pizer, 2016; Tummala-Narra, 2020, 2022). The Holmes Commission Report of the American Psychoanalytic Association (Holmes et al., 2024) has documented implicit and explicit racism experienced within American psychoanalytic institutions and called for action toward systemic racial recognition and healing. Still, questions concerning the extent to which racial minority experiences are mentalized within psychoanalysis remain.

Self-Disclosure and the Desire for Racial and Cultural Recognition

Over the past two decades, I have observed more people request a therapist of a similar racial and ethnic background, sexual orientation, gender, age, or some other aspect of social location and identity, in the hope of being understood and affirmed. In fact, recently, I received a request for a South Asian female therapist who understands neurodivergence and South Asian marriages. Such requests have been growing for several reasons. A person may have experienced discrimination within the therapeutic context (e.g., past therapy) and hopes for the recognition of traumatic and stressful experiences related to race and culture. They may fear that someone outside of their racial, ethnic, or religious group may pathologize them or their loved ones. More people are also hopeful about finding a therapist of a similar racial or ethnic background due to increased access to teletherapy. Perhaps even more significant for some patients is the specific targeting of people of minority status in the current political climate.

Most of my patients talk about the stress they feel related to policies attacking women's reproductive rights, immigrants, racial minorities, LGBTQ+ people, disabled people, and religious minorities, including a chronic sense of anxiety, demoralization, and helplessness. Others have wondered about my beliefs regarding the current U.S. president and political conflicts in Ukraine, the Middle East, and South Asia. The active collective traumas occurring within and outside the United States are no longer peripheral issues for patients but have rather become central concerns reflecting questions about safety, identity, belonging, and relationships. For many patients, it's imperative to know something about the therapist's social, cultural, and political perspectives, as it has become increasingly challenging to know whom to trust in a divisive sociopolitical climate. Furthermore, patients have access to at least some of the therapist's orientation toward social issues through the internet (e.g., Google searches and YouTube videos), leaving therapists with less anonymity (Richards, 2018).

There is also evidence that more therapists espouse a new sense of freedom in sharing relevant information regarding race and culture with patients, due to shifts in theoretical understandings of the therapeutic relationship (e.g., intersubjective and relational perspectives) and their own personal experiences of the sociopolitical climate. Interestingly, one study examining 268 therapists' views on political self-disclosure indicates that 87% of therapists discussed politics with their patients and that shared political views between the therapist and patient and therapists' political self-disclosure supported a stronger therapeutic alliance (Solomonov & Barber, 2019). Yet, serious questions remain regarding the determinants of such disclosures and their lasting impacts on therapeutic process, particularly when considering histories of colonization and slavery that mark American racial and cultural dynamics.

Bearing in mind theoretical understandings of self-disclosure mentioned earlier (Frankel, 2018; Richards, 2018; West, 2017), it is worth considering when self-disclosure regarding race and culture might be helpful to the patient and when it may disrupt the exploration of the patient's psychic material. For example, my Indian American patients have typically asked me early in our work together which part of India I am from, what Indian language I speak, and whether I was born in India or in the United States. These questions are ordinary yet important culturally affirming ways to introduce oneself to someone in the Indian context. In the U.S. therapeutic context, which is less familiar to most Indians and Indian Americans, direct responses to these questions are essential to building trust while also shaping a complex set of transferential reactions. By revealing that I am originally from Andhra Pradesh in South India, that I speak Telugu, and that I immigrated to the United States as a child, a patient may view me as someone who is familiar with India and Indian cultures. The patient may comment that they have been to Andhra Pradesh or know someone from there, or the patient might withhold expressing negative feelings about people from Andhra Pradesh or South India. Depending on the patient's history and circumstances, they may view my darker skin tone as less attractive, as light skin tones are often preferred among South Asians, or be relieved to work with a therapist who understands what it is like to have a darker skin tone. They may interpret my mainstream American accent as indicative of me as more Americanized and less in touch with my Indian heritage or, on the other hand, as indicative of someone who is able to better understand bicultural identity. They may wonder about my religious and spiritual life as they contemplate whether they can comfortably talk about their religion and spirituality with me. When I meet with patients who are not Indian or South Asian, similar questions arise, although there is less familiarity concerning racial, cultural, and religious experiences, heightening the possibility of a different set of conscious and unconscious stereotypes shaping their perceptions of me (Tummala-Narra, 2020, 2022). As such, any self-disclosure produces a tension for the patient to both know and not know me.

A poignant illustration of this tension of knowing and not knowing experienced by patients was provided by Grand (2014), a White analyst, who described her experience of meeting with her African American analyst who appeared White. After a few sessions, she learned from two other people that her therapist identified as an African American and that her analyst was a political activist in the past. Grand (2014, p. 234) reveals, "I knew that she thought I thought she was white. . . . What my analyst didn't know is that

I knew without asking. Discovering her racial identification from external sources, it was as if I had plundered Pandora's box. I had forbidden, extra-analytic knowledge. I had the puzzle of white skin, black identity. I had questions that had no place in classical psychoanalysis". In her moving account, Grand (2014, p. 239) describes her wish for a sense of sameness with her analyst: "I needed my analyst to be an intact Bubbie from Brooklyn. I was suffering from attachment trauma. I wanted a sense of sameness with my analyst, a sameness that was both familiar and safe". Grand (2014, p. 240) proceeds to share her dilemmas as the White patient who needed her African American analyst to be White due to a wish for an "intact maternal bond" and because of the enduring traumatic legacy of slavery rife with guilt and shame: "So, I passed my analyst, but I never forgot that she was African-American, and that she would not pass herself. In the folds of this paradox, I reenacted persecutory history; but I was also trying to resist, and repair this history. By knowing my analyst as an African-American woman who I could imagine as my white Bubbie, I trespassed on my analyst's subjectivity. But in the mad thicket of race, I was also creative and insistent: I wanted an intact, and inviolable, maternal shield" (Ibid, p. 240). By Grand's account, her analyst, through her empathic attunement became a transformational maternal shield.

Grand highlights the patient's fantasy of the therapist's race, which in the contemporary climate, is almost always influenced by what a patient learns online about the therapist prior to meeting the therapist. The therapist too fantasizes about the patient's race and culture and desires their own racial and cultural subjectivity to be recognized by the patient in some way (Pizer, 2016). Notably, while the decision to self-disclose must take into account how a patient may experience the therapist's disclosure based on the patient's specific history and circumstances, inadvertent and deliberate disclosures concerning race and culture can reflect the therapist's wish to be recognized as a cultural being. This is evident in the clothes or jewelry that the therapist wears and objects, such as artwork and furniture in their office or Zoom space.

Therapists' hope that they can have some significant aspects of their racial and cultural subjectivities be recognized by the patient can also communicate that race and culture are essential to the psyche and the therapeutic process. For example, one of my patients who is Brazilian American, after noticing a Ganesha statue in my office, asked me if I am a Hindu, to which I responded affirmatively. She then shared with me that she felt more comfortable telling me about her family's indigenous healing practices because she felt that Hindus, like other indigenous people, are also misunderstood or devalued in the dominant Judeo-Christian U.S. context. In retrospect, I realize that I wanted her to feel comfortable speaking with me about her spiritual beliefs. Perhaps by placing a Ganesha statue in my office, I also wished to reveal something about my Hindu spirituality, a significant part of my life, that is indeed largely misunderstood and devalued in the United States. Interestingly, in my own therapy, my White therapist displayed a small Ganesha statue in his office, which engendered a sense of hope that he may know something about Indian and Hindu culture and that perhaps I would not have to explain everything about being a Hindu to him. I imagine that he too wanted me to recognize him as a cultural being.

There are, of course, other ways that therapists convey their interest in race and culture, as evident in the questions we ask or how we respond verbally and nonverbally to the patient's experiences. Silence concerning issues of race and ethnicity, for instance, potentially conveys a disinterest in these issues, and therefore, in the core aspects of the psyche (Leary, 1997; Tummala-Narra, 2016). Silence can also indicate an unwillingness to delve into the complexity of racial and cultural dynamics in the therapeutic relationship. Furthermore, it is worth considering that what the patient and therapist present to each other is multiply determined (Akhtar, 2014; Holmes, 2012), such that race and culture are intertwined with other aspects of development and identity. Therefore, asking questions about a patient's history of immigration or experience of racism does not typically lead to discussions about immigration or race alone, but also about how they came to understand their heritage culture, family, and racial identifications.

Some self-disclosures are necessary for the recognition and deeper exploration of race and culture that move beyond superficial understandings of the patient's identity and social location. For example, my patient, Anthony, an African American man in his 40s, early in our work, shared with me that he is unsure about therapy as he was disappointed by a White therapist with whom he worked several years earlier. He said, "I feel like you would understand what it's like not to be White, but you still don't know what it's like to be Black. You're Indian or somewhere from South Asia, right?" I responded, "Yes, I'm Indian American. I came to the United States when I was young child. Can you say more about your concern about me not being Black?" Anthony stated, "I guess it would help for me to know that you will understand what it's like to be a minority in this country. You grew up here. So, I think you probably will get it". It was important for Anthony to know that I grew up primarily in the United States, as he proceeded, in subsequent sessions, to share experiences of racist bullying he faced since his early childhood. My self-disclosure alone was not sufficient for a deeper exploration of his racial trauma, but it helped him to secure a sense of safety, at least at the beginning stages of our work. The self-disclosure was followed by responding with curiosity and empathy when he talked about his anger, frustration, and helplessness about the racism he faces.

Reflecting on my countertransference, specifically making the distinction between his experiences of racism from mine, served as a guidepost to decisions about any further self-disclosures. This was especially important as I did not feel as though Anthony wanted me to share more details about my Indian American experiences but rather needed to know that my experiences were psychically somewhere near his. In some moments, he would say, "I feel like you get it. You don't say much about yourself, but I know you get it". These types of comments brought me to wonder about how best to secure his sense of trust in me and facilitate an inquiry into his own experiences without the intrusion of my own need for recognition of my racism-related pain. This is no simple task with Anthony or with any of my patients, as racial pain and loneliness (Suslovic, 2020) pose a silent but palpable strain on so many racial minority therapists who have been told in training or elsewhere to suppress their racial and cultural experiences in the name of therapeutic neutrality. While I believe Anthony benefitted from my self-disclosure and from my restraint in not disclosing further details about my experiences, other patients have benefited from knowing more details about me, such as the fact that I experience stereotypes based on gender, race, skin color, and religion similar to them, or that I have the experience of migrating to the United States from another country.

Self-Disclosure and Collective Trauma

Recent literature indicates that therapists may be more likely to inadvertently or deliberately self-disclose some personal details due to collective traumas, such as the COVID-19 pandemic and related death, illness, stress, and social and political strife and the use of technologies, such as Zoom (Brody, 2021; Luo et al., 2023). This is also true for active personal crises and traumas. Brody (2013) named the reality that there are no specific rules for self-disclosure under traumatic circumstances, specifically referring to disclosing her cancer diagnosis to her patients. She aptly recognizes how revealing her illness to her patients is intertwined with each patient's unique history. She states, "When an analyst self-discloses, it powerfully and suddenly activates an awareness of the analyst as separate. . . . Perhaps at such a moment, and in many moments after, we are triggering an enactment, the evocation of an unconscious connection to that time when the caretaker was first experienced as a separate person, a developmental process that provides the momentum for autonomy and connection" (Brody, 2013, p. 55). Here, Brody calls attention to the inevitability of self-disclosure under periods of crisis and trauma, and how self-disclosure brings to the foreground a patient's earlier separations, losses, and traumatic experiences.

Relatedly, past and present collective traumas (e.g., war, displacement, sexual violence, policies regarding immigration, reproductive rights, and LGBTQ+ rights) faced by both patients and therapists are felt in therapeutic work, regardless of whether they are being explicitly discussed (Dorozhkin, 2023; Holmes, 2012; Mukha, 2025). For instance, Dorozhkin (2023), a Ukrainian psychoanalytic therapist, has written about how Ukrainian therapists have had to change the typical therapeutic frame in the face of the Russian invasion, and offer support to patients through phone calls, emails, inviting them to share housing with them, and providing information to help secure physical safety. In this case, self-disclosures were both unavoidable and in fact, therapists are "encouraged to speak as citizens of their country" (Dorozhkin, 2023, p. 248). In my own work, as that of many other therapists over the past decade in the United States, I have helped patients develop safety plans in the face of potential deportation of family members. The climate of fear in which we conduct our work calls for active recognition of racism and xenophobia and at times, direct assistance for patients to secure basic safety.

Seligman (2021, p. 121) has written about political countertransference, closely related to race- and ethnicity-related countertransference, where he highlighted the feelings of uncertainty, powerlessness, and fear that he shares with his patients with regard to the current sociopolitical climate in the United States. He stated, "When patients talk about how appalled they are about the detention of young children in cages or how scared they are of COVID, it's easy to sympathize. What's different about these moments, though, is that I often feel a quite similar feeling, and I frequently respond from my position as a citizen, rather than my 'analytic role'". Seligman's sentiments call into question what the "analytic role" looks like amidst collective trauma. Specifically, the therapist is tasked with the challenge of recognizing both the harmful realities of collective trauma and the potential for splitting where the therapist and patient collude in an us-them position that diminishes empathy and avoids inquiry into the patient's and the therapist's own aggression.

While it is true that the current sociopolitical climate has marked new dilemmas regarding self-disclosure concerning collective traumas, for most racial minorities, such dilemmas are not new, as we have had little choice regarding our racial positioning within U.S. society. We have experienced racism, xenophobia, and sexism, among many other forms of exclusion and discrimination. Intergenerational traumas rooted in slavery, genocide, and colonization live inside us, and we have been implicitly and explicitly asked to remain silent about these experiences within our therapeutic work. We have theoretical differences regarding self-disclosure and we, like our patients, are concerned about the legitimacy of our own racial pain within institutional settings. Many of us have not had the benefit of exploring our own sociocultural traumas within our analysis or therapy due to the analyst's or therapist's reluctance to engage with these issues. As such, the denial and minimization of our own sociocultural traumas leave us feeling unsure about self-disclosure with our patients. And yet, we know the importance of recognizing our racial and cultural backgrounds with our patients.

In my own work, the issue of intergenerational sociocultural trauma endured by my patients is ubiquitous, spanning internalized stereotypes to violence based on race, ethnicity, national origin, gender, religion, sexuality, and disability. The legacies of these traumas within my own life intersect with that of my clients, as I consider questions regarding self-disclosure. I am often left uncertain about what the long-term impacts of my self-disclosure or non-self-disclosure might be for my patients, as our shared and separate histories are shaped by complex layers of social, family, and personality dynamics. The present sociopolitical climate triggers old and new anxieties about loss, separation, and belonging.

For instance, my patient, Shivani, a second-generation Indian American woman in her 40s, a year into our work, shared with me a memory of Partition (India and Pakistan) passed on to her by her grandfather. Shivani expresses, "My grandfather was always so angry. It was so hard to be around him. But then, I think about his suffering. He was a child when he was forced to move in the Partition. He told me just once and then never talked about it again. I'm just left with holes in these stories. I haven't thought about this in years". Shivani proceeded to tell me how much she longed to know more about her family's history, one that is marked by repeated displacements from one part of India to another and then across multiple countries. She wanted to know more about how British colonization impacted her family, a topic that her parents and grandparents had refused to talk about. It is no coincidence that she is reminded of the Partition of India as she is terrified by the racist targeting of immigrants and the mass displacement of people across the world. She shared, "I thought this (U.S.) would always be my home, but maybe I will be forced to move just like when I was little and how my grandparents had to leave their homes. I feel like I'm reduced to my skin color here. Nothing I've done here or for the people here matters. In India, it was the British and Hindus and Muslims. Here, it is just our skin color". I resonated with Shivani's grief, and when she asked me if I could relate to what she shared, I responded, "Yes, I'm feeling disappointed and scared too". She said, "I needed to hear that. I'm not alone. Thank you".

Yet, there were other moments when Shivani shared her political views on Narendra Modi's discriminatory policies against Muslims in India. She stated, "I don't want to carry my grandparents' wounds into how I think about Muslims. They (Muslims and Hindus) are all misguided, this fighting over religion supposedly. I don't want to judge people like my grandparents and my parents". I empathized with Shivani's sadness, fear, and loss, and I chose not to talk about my own family's history of being victimized by political violence in India, even though some part of me wanted her to know and communicate to her that I too have painful feelings about British colonization and Partition. I remain uncertain as to whether I would have disclosed anything about my history if she would have asked me directly. Perhaps, I felt safer in sharing in her racialized pain in the United States than in the Partition-related grief, as we both have holes in fully knowing our family histories in India. I have wondered whether my self-disclosure about politics in the United States or in India could help Shivani deepen her understanding of her feelings about the religious and political polarization underlying Partition and the current political polarization of the United States, both of which have important implications for her connection to and differentiation from her family. At the same time, I wonder if my self-disclosure could potentially fuel a reproduction of the splitting dynamics, characterizing her family and the broader social environment, that she is seeking to resolve. Perhaps, I would feel differently about my self-disclosure with her at a different historical moment.

Concluding Thoughts

The decision to self-disclose regarding race and culture in psychotherapy requires a careful exploration of multiple determinants of the patient's and therapist's life histories and present circumstances and realities. Self-disclosure dilemmas faced by therapists reflect the paradoxical hypervisibility and invisibility of race and culture in the United States. A pluralistic approach, considering all psychoanalytic perspectives (Holmes, 2012), is needed to appreciate the complexity of the meanings of race and culture for each patient and each therapist. Notably, the subjectivity and external realities of racial minority therapists are distinct with important implications for transference and countertransference. While psychoanalysis has historically ignored the significance of race and culture in conceptualizations of neutrality and self-disclosure, the growing awareness of race and culture in contemporary psychoanalysis and heightened sociopolitical stress call for further attention to the role of self-disclosure in either expanding and deepening inquiry of the self, inhibiting such inquiry, or both.

References

Akhtar, S. (2014). Psychoanalytic treatment of trauma and the analyst's personality. *Psychoanalytic Inquiry, 34*(3), 204–213. https://doi.org/10.1080/07351690.2014.889468
Balint, M. (1968). *The basic fault: Therapeutic aspects of regression*. London & New York: Tavistock Publications.
Brody, S. R. (2013). Entering night country: Reflections on self-disclosure and vulnerability. *Psychoanalytic Dialogues, 23*(1), 45–58. https://doi.org/10.1080/10481885.2013.752703
Brody, S. R. (2021). Facing the facts: Self-disclosure and the analytic relationship swimming in dark places. *American Imago, 78*(3), 485–490. https://dx.doi.org/10.1353/aim.2021.0023
Bromberg, P. M. (2010). Minding the dissociative gap. *Contemporary Psychoanalysis, 46*(1), 19–31. https://doi.org/10.1080/00107530.2010.10746037
Comas-Díaz, L., & Jacobsen, F. M. (1991). Ethnocultural transference and countertransference in the therapeutic dyad. *The American Journal of Orthopsychiatry, 61*(3), 392–402. https://doi.org/10.1037/h0079267
Dorozhkin, V. (2023). Therapeutic relationships in wartime Ukraine. *Psychoanalytic Psychology, 40*(4), 247–250. https://doi.org/10.1037/pap0000482
Frankel, J. (2018). Thoughts on the limits of a mutual technique. *American Journal of Psychoanalysis, 78*(4), 350–360. https://doi.org/10.1057/s11231-018-9157-2
Grand, S. (2014). Skin memories: On race, love and loss. *Psychoanalysis, Culture and Society, 19*(3), 232–249.
Holmes, D. E. (2012). Racial transference reactions in psychoanalytic treatment: An update. In S. Akhtar (Ed.), *The African American experience: Psychoanalytic perspectives* (pp. 363–376). Jason Aronson.
Holmes, D. E., Hart, A. H., Powell, D. R., Stoute, B. J., Chodorow, N. J., Davids, M. F., Dennis, E., Glover, W., González, F. J., Hamer, F. M., Javier, R. Art., Katz, M., Leary, K. R., Maree, R. D., Méndez, T., Moskowitz, M., Moss, D., Tummala-Narra, P., Ueng-McHale, J., . . . McNamara, S. (2024). In pursuit of racial equality in American Psychoanalysis: Findings and recommendations from the Holmes Commission. *Journal of the American Psychoanalytic Association, 72*(3), 407–552. https://doi.org/10.1177/00030651241253623

Leary, K. (1997). Race, self-disclosure, and 'forbidden talk': Race and ethnicity in contemporary clinical practice. *The Psychoanalytic Quarterly*, *66*(2), 163–189. https://doi.org/10.1080/21674086.1997.11927530

Luo, X., Aafjes-van Doorn, K., Békés, V., Prout, T. A., & Hoffman, L. (2023). Therapist self-disclosure in teletherapy early in the COVID-19 pandemic: Associations with real relationship and traumatic distress. *Clinical Psychology & Psychotherapy*. https://doi.org/10.1002/cpp.2915

Mitchell, S. A. (1988). *Relational concepts in psychoanalysis: An integration*. Harvard University Press.

Mukha, O. (2025). Subjectivity in therapy during war. *Psychoanalytic Dialogues*, *35*(2), 273–274. https://doi.org/10.1080/10481885.2025.2471255

Pizer, A. S. (2016). Do I have to tell my patients I'm blind? *Psychoanalytic Perspectives, 13*, 214–229. https://doi.org/10.1080/1551806X.2016.1156435

Richards, A. (2018). Some thoughts on self-disclosure. *Psychoanalytic Review*, *105*(2), 137–156. https://doi.org/10.1521/prev.2018.105.2.137

Seligman, S. (2021). Disturbing positions: The crisis and potentials of sociopolitical emotions. *Psychoanalytic Psychology*, *38*(2), 120–122. https://doi.org/10.1037/pap0000346

Solomonov, N., & Barber, J. P. (2019). Conducting psychotherapy in the Trump era: Therapists' perspectives on political self-disclosure, the therapeutic alliance, and politics in the therapy room. *Journal of Clinical Psychology*, *75*(9), 1508–1518. https://doi.org/10.1002/jclp.22801

Stolorow, R. D. (1988). Intersubjectivity, psychoanalytic knowing, and reality. *Contemporary Psychoanalysis*, *24*(2), 331–338. https://doi.org/10.1080/00107530.1988.10746247

Suslovic, B. (2020). Mitigating racial loneliness as transformative psychoanalytic work. *Psychoanalysis, Culture & Society*, *25*(3), 480–489. https://doi.org/10.1057/s41282-020-00175-4

Tummala-Narra, P. (2016). *Psychoanalytic theory and cultural competence in psychotherapy*. American Psychological Association. https://doi.org/10.1037/14800-000

Tummala-Narra, P. (2020). The fear of immigrants. *Psychoanalytic Psychology*, *37*(1), 50–61. https://doi.org/10.1037/pap0000245

Tummala-Narra, P. (2022). Can we decolonize psychoanalytic theory and practice? *Psychoanalytic Dialogues*, *32*(3), 217–234. https://doi.org/10.1080/10481885.2022.2058326

West, M. (2017). Self-disclosure, trauma and the pressures on the analyst. *Journal of Analytical Psychology*, *62*(4), 585–601. https://doi.org/10.1111/1468-5922.12338

Section 3

Transparency and Porous Boundaries

Chapters by S. Brody, A. Adelman, and K. Starr

Over the past ten years a series of extraordinary external events has challenged theoretical concepts surrounding the meaning and necessity of self-disclosure in the practice of individual psychotherapy and psychoanalysis. Presidential elections, a divisive population, together with the global pandemic, have dramatically affected the consulting room process. In our dyadic spaces we have met our clients, sometimes for the first time, in a two-dimensional platform. We notice that the clinical boundary is porous and, concretely, transparent. The spaces that were only imagined are visible. Though we sometimes cloud the background of our workspaces, our clients know that we are home. Similarly, we see our clients in their homes, spaces that we had usually imagined, or sometimes never reflected upon. Bedrooms, bathrooms, kitchens. Children walk through doors, partners say hello. Intrusions can include marital tension, the sudden muting of the interaction due to a phone call or request. Cars offer privacy, and escape, but are suddenly perilous when driven during sessions.

Though we create protection through distance, we are simultaneously navigating an activated and polarized social and political field. Discussions of identity, misogyny, harassment, activism and personal attacks, racism and climate anxiety, have led many conversations to include the political. The criteria for treatment are not about education and experience alone, but can include political party, religious beliefs, or social status. Requesting information about affiliation has not often been a question at the beginning of a treatment, until now. Resistance to an answer, or the wrong answer, can sometimes be a deal breaker. Core themes in our work – vulnerability, anxiety, hopelessness – have become bound to the external in a new way. The window into the personal is more accessible. The media onslaught of constant breaking news alerts, tweets and threats, political decisions and challenges create a frequency of high-intensity moments. These external triggers are wrapped around relationship dynamics, traumas, and affect. Protest, longings for consolation, and reactions to social action (or inaction) have also emerged. The political and social have merged with the analytic landscape in a way that I cannot remember. Maintaining clinical curiosity, empathy, and neutrality in this turbulent context can be deeply challenging.

DOI: 10.4324/9781003584803-10

In the following chapters, each author describes the personal and the upheaval, bearing up through the onslaught. My own piece, originally written during the pandemic, describes the transition to the virtual platform, the encroachment of the unexpected under forced quarantine, and the many clinical contradictions that ensue as we confront the lethality of the COVID virus. It offers a post-COVID reflection on what has changed, and what hasn't. Anne Adelman shows her flexibility and responsiveness to the opportunities that might be therapeutically utilized in the unique time frame of the pandemic. She reveals how she was able to use the virtual platform, inside and outside, allowing unexpected guests and landscapes, and a steady attunement within the changing dynamics. Karen E. Starr shows what can happen when analytic curiosity and empathy collide with political alliances and expectations, leading to unexpected disclosures, demands, and negotiations. In each case, we learn more about the challenges to "the frame", to analytic neutrality, and to the management of countertransference feelings. Though these are examples of a specific time, each represents the challenge of external intrusion and the way these external events exert a powerful influence on the therapeutic work and the visibility of the analyst's identity.

7 Quarantine

Swimming in Dark Places[1]

Stephanie R. Brody

Quarantine

Today I found an open door to a forgotten place. Searching through my digital archive for a lost document, I noticed a file – *Day One* – that caught my attention. Intrigued, I clicked. *Day One Coronavirus Self-Quarantine*.

A diary.

There, a lost record opened to a time, the unsettling early moments of exposure and separation. Palpable anxiety. How quickly we forget what happened, what we did, and how vulnerable we felt.

March 13, 2020

Everything is the same and everything is different. I am still yelling at the radio when Trump blames the Obama administration. It has been torturous to make the decision to limit contact with my patients by shifting to the phone or online platforms. I know it will be awkward and challenging for some who have not utilized this form of connection before. It is for me as well. I risk losing the intimacy with individuals who require face-to-face, real time, to build a relationship. I will lose the nuances that are available when I share the space in my office. It is challenging to understand some of my colleagues who have elected to continue seeing patients in person, as though they are immune to the virus, and don't need to follow the restrictions.

In the day-to-day life, there are questions about the normal activities. What does everyday life mean now? My doctor advises that my decision to work remotely is correct, but there is the ominous warning that there is no way that this virus will not, at some point, penetrate my body and affect my health. I go swimming in the chlorinated pool, avoiding contact with people as I plunge. Entering the almost empty space, liquid enters my mouth, nose, ears, my eyes. It's not a question of if, but when.

Day 2, March 14

I have made a decision to avoid the gym after speaking with friends who have family members in the research field. The virus can survive on plastic and

DOI: 10.4324/9781003584803-11

stainless steel. It would be impossible to wipe down all surfaces of the common bathroom area, the bannisters, doorknobs, the shower. Some are still meeting patients in their offices.

I begin the process of contacting patients and hear the genuine relief that we will be meeting remotely. Many of them, health care providers themselves, have also been told to work from home if they do not provide inpatient care. As my Monday schedule begins to materialize, I see that my day is full.

More problematic is the disruption of my routine. Without a swim, without the rhythmic breathing and peaceful solitude, I could lose my bearing. My body is feeling stiff and my knee hurts. Being outside for a walk on a beautiful day, with my friend at a safe distance, feels almost normal, but should we be even this close? I notice that my house feels cluttered and as the day goes on, I realize how I will need to prepare a new office that feels peaceful and offers me the comfort to provide care to my patients.

Day 3, March 15

Irritability begins in earnest. Disease/Death/Divorce? How will we contain ourselves as we respond to the containment rules? My friend's adult child is sent home from work – likely exposed. What to do with her young child and her recently hospitalized spouse? Patients are beginning to call with eruptions of anxiety – attacks of fear based on exposure and previous catastrophic expectations. We are all in the same boat.

One genuinely remarkable gem, in a day of chaos: Joyce DiDonato. The opera singer alerts her fans that she will be live-streaming excerpts of *Werther*, the opera that she was supposed to premiere at the Met this week that I would have seen in person. It is thrilling to watch her, with tenor Piotr Beczala, create the opera in her living room. Thousands, from all over the world, view this amazing and epic display of art and generosity; I am filled with gratitude and humility for this unlikely gift. It is an expression of deep humanity in a back fill of the garbage and venom that has been lately spewing from others who have been emboldened to argue that what is happening to us is a hoax.

Day 4, March 16

First day of seeing patients online and by phone.

Coronavirus is a Rorschach test.

My doctor patients express dread, dread about decisions, about exposure. They are enraged by the absence of efforts to protect and provide adequate services. They are fearful that they will bring illness home to their families. Another patient describes "liberation": rules are abandoned because "we're all going to die". She rejects all efforts at social isolation, or any awareness of a larger impact on the community, a form of self-destructiveness that recreates a history of family rebellion. Another patient reports an opening of deeper feelings, a desire for intimacy, a sense of clarity regarding personal relationships: "if there were only one person I could be with during this time, who would that be?"

I am fumbling with technology and my new phone. One snowy day can be managed, but what if this form of treatment goes on for days, weeks, months?

Day 5, March 17

Continued transition into telehealth. Agitated patients. There is a remarkable absence of awareness regarding the level of contamination potential. Patients in group housing describe individuals "in quarantine" that are sharing common spaces. There seems little awareness of how contamination can spread, or how one quarantine really means self-quarantine for others. What is my role as a therapist in this situation? Is it therapeutic to intervene, assert what limited knowledge of information I have received from a caretaker who seems uninformed?

Taking a walk. Encountering more people along my path – avoid eye contact, but also swerving to avoid physical contact. It is awkward to ask for distance.

My nightly balm is the Met opera screening on my computer. Last night, *La Boheme*.

Day 6, March 18

Walking as best I can. It's taking a toll on my knee – not to swim. Working with patients doing telehealth is interesting and different, each day. Challenging in some ways – I'm learning to use the speaker and Zoom and it helps, but it's hard on the vocal cords. Patients seem receptive – mostly. Ambivalence, depending on the person involved. More distance.

I walked to my office today to retrieve the mail and was horrified to see a few people there. The rest of the building is shut down – no one else in the office, including the local Minuteman press.

The nightly opera stream from the Met is immensely soothing, but it is hard to do anything else. My office has never been in my home, so unlike some colleagues, I miss having space between work and home. It feels like I'm always at work or getting ready for work.

The diary stops after six days.

My effort to document an eerie new experience that I thought would be worth remembering someday, ends after barely one week. It was a time when the veil between spaces was altered, when access changed. When the emergency was all encompassing, and we waited to find out who would survive. I wrote of that time, of my effort to reach into my words for a stabilizing comfort. It seems long ago, like a strange dream. But we all went through it together. That first year of quarantine challenged the frame, the many theories of self-disclosure that we trusted within the analytic praxis. In quarantine, we disclosed and were exposed. We made keyholes to look through, and were telescoped into other worlds. It was a year like none other. The following narrative collapses that time, though it would continue beyond this chapter. Here is a year in COVID world.

Living With the Virus: Present Tense[2]

Every day, simply showing up in the rectangular frame has been an act of disclosure. A convergence of viral, political, racial, and personal – on both sides of the screen. In past times, disclosure has been about intrusion, deliberate, accidental . . . the inevitable; life events, medical diagnoses, losses and personal grenades that can impact our work. Each, forms of disclosure and dyadic reckonings, repairs and opportunities, have also been stories that raise our awareness and have set the stage for other possibilities. But this year has been a different kind of year. Unanticipated. Unprecedented. So many, most of us in the clinical world have had the privilege of working, but all of us have had to weather the hard knock of encroaching reality. The norms that we took for granted, as individuals, as a society, and as a country have been altered. What it is like to work in this new reality? This is a story in and out of time, in and out of ourselves, grappling with the shared realities, the familiarity and the strangeness of it, and to consider how we will be wrestling with it for years to come. Three months later, after summer arrives, we contend with the growing awareness that this interruption will go on for a long time. Dealing with the ongoing limitations brings about the embrace of a new landscape – Zoom is an unexpected accommodation, but not the only one. Before the onset of COVID, swimming has been a daily activity. But in a pandemic, even a chlorinated pool holds danger. I am fortunate that Walden Pond is only ten minutes from home.

Even on a very sunny day in late May, it is too soon for the pond. But I can no longer wait for 78-degree chlorinated pool water. Without a wetsuit, I try to ignore the icy water covering my feet, ankles, knees and plunge in. After months of interruption, the physical shock of freezing water causes my muscles to seize up. After several strokes, when my heart starts to race, and I gulp for air, I realize that I have stopped breathing. I remind myself to open my lungs. Reengaged by the benefits of oxygen, the rest of me kicks in – arms and legs restored and mobilized. My body remembers. It is a short swim in unknown territory. Over many more days, the air warms and the pond absorbs the sun; the water is an unexpected source of reliability, comfort and surprise. At first, I swim near the shoreline where it is shallow, where I can stand, if necessary, grounded. Walden Pond is a kettle hole, created by a receding ice age. 108 feet deep, the sharp drops challenge the inexperienced swimmer. Busy summer traffic reveals the progression of numerous swimmers attached to neon orange, green and yellow floating buoys – a signal that the 62-acre space can swallow up anyone who suffers a cramp far from shore.

But as the summer continues, as I became more familiar, I am more confident, and curious about the dark spaces. Just as in my work, the hard constriction of the space, is becoming familiar. And new forms of communication – unplanned, never before included, are part of the territory.

Back home, the daily convergence of personal space with professional life is disorienting. The transition from my home to my office is not only geographical but also internal. I situate myself so that my computer screen bisects the new office space, a pseudo barrier to my line of sight to set up the *new selfie*. The background – a still life in a frame changes depending on the time of day, or the weather: back light, a view of trees, or a black rectangle after sundown. The mural. And there is no getting away from that first mirror image moment. I am quick to "pin" my patient (a term that evokes a slew of butterfly associations – from opera to museum exhibits) and make myself into a postage stamp or better – eliminate myself entirely from the screen. How does this matter? What does this effort mean about who I am as an analyst, what am I trying to convey, or hide?

Screen to Screen. Quarantine to Quarantine

"Dr. Brody, is that a painting behind you?".

My patient is wondering about the mural that my mother painted to cover the drab closet doors that extend over an entire wall. It is a vibrant landscape of orange, reds, and green. I like having it as my scenic backdrop.

I smile and say: "It's a mural".

She says: "I miss being in your office. This is not the same".

Using Zoom for the first time on his last day working with me, the perpetual scowl of this older man turns into a broad smile, an expression I have never seen.

"My mother was the only one who liked to paint using colors that clash. It's good to see them. It will be a nice memory to take with me. That's enough. I don't want to talk anymore".

What is behind, within, or between the screen, is penetrated. It is one of the liabilities of our reliance on social media platforms. We make decisions about what to share in our separate worlds – some are revealed, others remain hidden. But collisions are inevitable.

Amid growing political tensions, a patient has been tracking a colleague's Facebook posts – information that might have been inadvertently exposed or incautiously hidden. Triggered and decompensating, his reaction, full of profanities and ominous messages, is broadcast to the clinical staff. The screen may appear protective, but murderous impulses and threats reveal a hidden risk. Perhaps safety is an illusion. Can treatment continue under these circumstances? I am only intermittently capable of reining in my astonishment when my single patients ignore their vulnerability to COVID, and abandon quarantines and masks. Hungry for contact, the wish to find a partner suddenly descends on a patient who sees her reproductive potential dwindling over the prolonged retreat from human contact. Scouring dating sites, she meets up with strangers, hoping to secure a partner, or at least a respite from loneliness.

Face to face with the intensity of their need, a delusional sense of immunity and a flouting of risk emerges. My disbelief rises. In touch with my wish to break through denial, I struggle with my wish to force reality into the room and penetrate the protective lid of omnipotence. Fear and vulnerability have gone missing, at least consciously, and I have been drawn into judgment, criticism and disbelief. This is another threat – the potential collapse of curiosity and exploration. In this dangerous time, I struggle to grapple with the intrusion of an unprecedented reality and find that for some people, there is satisfaction in the power to exert life-threatening harm through the willful exposure of another person. I feel responsible for this reckless behavior, for the other people who will be exposed; how is this different from past enactments and dangerous behavior? Self-reflection regarding the concept of "personal responsibility", aggression, or the possibility of unprocessed anger, appears out of reach. Trolling for sexual contact, an enactment that is especially risky, remains robust despite my analytic efforts. My thoughts are drawn to the other thousands in our country who defy, deny, or minimize the risks to themselves or others. Does this rebellion represent a profound wish for contact, and need for intimacy, or is this personal aggression? Is this a denial of death?

Essential workers have no choice and need the money. Terrified of losing their jobs, they show up, masked, to diligently pack bags, arrange pastries, and make deliveries. They arrive home after long shifts, waiting for the virus to strike. Flooded with the anguish for my patients who work in health care, I think about how overwhelmed and dispirited they have become. The initial terror and risk have subsided into a numbness, indistinguishable from detachment and dissociation. Forced to cover themselves in protective gear at work, they strip down before going home. Increasingly paranoid about exposing others, they sleep in basements, or never go home at all. The isolation is profound and traumatizing. Each relationship becomes an opportunity to communicate frustration, fear, and personal agony as we dive into the darkness of the soul.

I work in the safety of my home, wondering when we will explore the imbalance of my privilege as I continue to receive referrals, send invoices, and practice my trade. We situate ourselves in these high-tech frames to maintain our safety from the unsparing virus – we work this way to change the odds – to keep illness and mortality at bay. After almost a year of practicing this way, we don't really talk about how we're getting used to it and what this acceptance means. The unstable Wi-Fi, the eye fatigue, the benefits of the 30-second commute. Precious minutes are newly available and entice with possibility, but jolt with unavoidable limitations. I am knocked back by the awareness. So obvious it's like a slap in the face – that we are all avoiding – the vulnerability. The pervasive fog of loss that descends on us as we hear daily death statistics alongside the increasing awareness that this restriction will not be changing soon. We adapt and adjust, but do we speak of what we share? It's right there. Because my mind often moves to the forces of time, the slipping through of hourglass sand as we remain tightly enclosed in our spaces, the pandemic symbolizes an encroaching darkness. We are separate because, through the transparent screen of disclosure and non-disclosure, we can see each other's mortality.

How do we make the most of what we have, within the limitations of this time? Is it possible to live life to the fullest with the walls closing in? I see patients, young and old, facing the facts for first time – the recognition of our existential fate – and it hits with a resounding crack. On an episode of Fresh Air, Terry Gross interviews Marielle Heller, the director of "A Beautiful Day in the Neighborhood" (Fresh Air, November 20, 2019). It is a film about a journalist who uncovers the heroic in Fred Rogers. When Ms. Heller lets her 3-year-old view "the famous Fish Episode" when Fred Rogers introduces death to children, she feels a sense of dread. She watches and waits, as understanding and grief sweep over her son. It is searing. As a parent, there is nothing else to do but cry with her son, as they weep together over what we all must bear.

Because my work, my writing and my exploration has often led me to this place, I like to think I'm ready when this awareness arrives. I signal that I am open to bearing the grief and the challenge with my patients, to guide and understand them in our shared mortal fate. One thing I have learned from my immersion in this topic is how much can be changed – what is possible to control – and what cannot. It is one of the greatest ordeals that we must regularly accept our helplessness, to mourn what cannot be changed and to go on. It is, after all, one of our great assets that we can bear this entirely human of challenges.

Such is the life's blood of our work as psychoanalysts. The different stories – what moves into the foreground of our minds, of our work and of our worlds. What do we decide to quarantine, and what is brought into the light, and how different dilemmas and personal forces exert their influence. Our special burdens include shepherding our patients through the moments of darkness and despair. There is something especially profound to me, as we leave this extraordinarily challenging year behind. The great losses, the political turmoil, the reckonings with racial justice, that will become encoded in a shared historical memory. The pieces of a newly formed Zoom world are to be embedded in a casing like no other we have recently experienced. A time capsule. But unlike the hard bottom surface of the swimming pool that is tabooed for fear of viral exposure, the underground of the pond is elusive in the changing light. Day after day, engaged with the now familiar rock cropping, protruding branches, and lake weeds, the water transforms into liquid scaffolding. The air inside me and around me is fuel. The depth revealed in the dark space that opened beneath as the sandy bottom fell away. At first, I shied away from all of that was dark and unseen. But then, I noticed my comfort in the depth. There is rhythm in the action, and the security of the water's comforting support. As the pond changes in the light, the swims are longer, each stroke affirming my relationship to the larger containing body. The dark underground tells me that there is no way to touchdown, and now, each plunge moves me from the wide spread of eternity to an unexpected freedom. It is magical. Clearly, there is something in that water.

This is the unknown and unknowable that becomes the known, the understandable, the surprise in what is continuous and what is evolving. The edges of the kettle hole are like the imposition of our clocks, the edges of our working space. There are the recognizable outcroppings that establish landmarks, and the navigational tools when we are lost or obscured. We name the destinations Thoreau's Cove, The Ice Quarry, transference, enactment, free association – and the shared vocabulary that tells us where we have travelled and what may be revealed on the far shore, if we are willing to go there.

In 1854, Henry David Thoreau wrote about his self-imposed two-year quarantine – to a small cabin in Concord Massachusetts. He said:

> *I went to the woods because I wished to live deliberately, to front only the essential facts of life, and see if I could not learn what it had to teach, and not, when I came to die, discover that I had not lived.*
>
> – Henry David Thoreau, *Walden* (1996 [1854])

Eventually even that which feels too dark or deep becomes familiar. This is when we can swim, stroke to stroke in the deep kettle pond of life, in the singular emotional pods that we make in our day-to-day clinical life. This is where the facts of our existence play in the light of the everyday and entice us out of the safety of the shallow end. We are quarantined and exposed. Protected and vulnerable. We can be seen and are seen through.

Epilogue 2025: Quarantine Reflection

What did it mean, to grasp the threads of longing and reconciliation from the watery deep so long ago? I went to the pond for exercise, to locate the rhythm of my body so reliant on routine, now separated from so much that was normal: A broad landscape restricted by the compelling forces of loss and anxiety. The imminence of death fashioned in harrowing statistics, multiplied by the maddening fatal chirps of bluster and incompetence. That awful soundscape returns now, the overwhelming din of revenge, cruelty, and loss. There is no getting away from the outright disclosures of aggression, power and hatred that are expressed in the handcuffs, abductions, and bullets. The noise carries across borders. The two-dimensional screen is utilized, not only as a protection, but also serves to disseminate falsehoods, unfettered by fact checks. Indifference is a false form of quarantine that does not fortify the boundaries. We are at risk again of an undoing, though the context of *this* illness, the nature of *this* viral spread, is more toxic when there are no new vaccines to curb its damage.

The summer of 2020 will stand out as a unique time and space. My feet, so unused to the rocky bottom, now navigate the depth with ease. The kettle hole is a reference point, a way back to memory and dark discovery; filtered with light and movements of the deep inhabitants, its presence mesmerizes and reveals the hidden spaces, newly arrived. Back in the office, "virtual" space has become an option for everyday psychotherapy, no longer reserved for snow days, or pandemics. The art that covers the walls of my official workplace represent a combination of evocative landscape, color and imagination. The objects on my windowsill, a marble egg, a miner's lamp, an hourglass have been selected for personal meaning. Though visible every day, they are only occasionally mentioned. The absence of curiosity and regard for the symbols that hold iconic meaning for me – light in the darkness, the passage of time, the source of life – remain a steady presence, a point of reference, an emotional compass. My clients read the book spines or gaze out the window as they lie on the couch. We have escaped the quarantine and indulge in the commonplace exploration of disclosure and non-disclosure, of knowing and not-knowing. Of here and gone.

And here again.

Notes

1 Copyright © 2021 Johns Hopkins University Press. A version of this article first appeared in American Imago, Volume 78, Number 3, Fall 2021 as Facing the Facts: Self Disclosure and the Analytic Relationship; Swimming in Dark Places. Published with permission by Johns Hopkins University Press.

2 The following narrative includes a version of a talk originally presented at the Annual Meeting of the American Psychoanalytic Association, February 2021. Sections were previously published in American Imago, Vol. 78, No. 3, 485–490.

References

Fresh Air NPR November 20, 2019 'Beautiful Day' Director on Mister Rogers' 'Radical Notion': Telling Kids The Truth.

Thoreau, H. D. (1996 [1854]). *Walden*. New York: Book of the Month Club.

8 Being Apart Together

The Virtual Landscape in Psychoanalysis

Anne Adelman

Growing up in New York City, I often caught glimpses of other people's lives through the rows of windows that faced the windows of my family's apartment. From our kitchen window, I could look down a broad air shaft, to the rear courtyard of my building. Across the way and to the left, dainty curtains hung above the small table where an old lady sometimes sat, alone, sipping tea. Above her and to the right, a child peered through safety bars, clutching the ears of a stuffed bunny. The large living room window of our apartment looked out over the New York cityscape, my elementary school in the foreground, the landscape spreading out past the Empire State building and, beyond, to the former World Trade Towers. On sick days, I would look down wistfully through my bedroom window into the windows of my school and watch insect-sized children, their little forms moving around the part of the classroom that was within my line of sight. How strange to see into a world – *my world!* – from the outside looking in, as things buzzed along without me, visible proof that I was not the center of the world I inhabited.

These glimpses allowed me to tell myself stories about the other denizens of the city, reassuring me that I was not alone. New York fairly teemed with signs of the private lives of others, details that were invisible when I walked along the sidewalks, outdoors, amid the maze of tall buildings.

The Zoom world, where our patients' images pop open onto our screen like jack-in-the boxes, brings to mind these moments from my childhood – what I saw of other people's dwellings through their tiny windows – where peeks of other people's lives connected me to the rest of humanity and offered an escape from the confined spaces of my own four walls.

I was curious about what glimpses of my patients' lives I would capture through their Zoom screens. Could I peek around the corner of the screen, into a previously invisible space, outside of, and off limits to, the analytic frame?

I have a patient who is fond of saying, whenever he steps across the threshold into my office, "This is your house. If I do anything wrong, you can make me leave. You run the show here, you're in charge". At the beginning of the pandemic, this patient was reluctant to meet via Zoom or FaceTime, so we met by phone for a while. However, as loneliness and isolation pressed down more intensely, the patient asked to meet via Zoom after all.

DOI: 10.4324/9781003584803-12

At the first Zoom meeting, I couldn't help but think to myself, "Now we're in *your* house. You can hang up anytime. You can show me what you want me to see and keep the rest under wraps". I saw, as I looked around, certain objects that the patient had spoken about over the years: a piece of art, a leather chair, a book on a carved wooden stand. I had the strange impression of somehow looking too intently – gazing into the screen and watching the signs of life reflected back at me, the wagging eyebrows, the nerve twitching above an eyelid, the lips readying to form a word.

Of course, my patients shared my curiosity. They, too, wished to step beyond the confines of what the screen permits. "Are those walls blue?" one person asks, although it is clear they can see the color of the wall behind me. "Is that a seashell above the doorway, over there?" "Are you in front of a window? What are you facing?" Earlier in the summer, my neighbor's rooster had the habit of cock-a-doodling at all hours of the day, which brought my patients merriment and glee, some confusion notwithstanding – "Are you on a farm?" to which I'd reply that no, residents of my neighborhood are permitted to keep chickens in the backyard.

At the beginning, it was a fact we faced together – that we are united in this moment, that we all experience the same strange conditions of being in this pandemic. For some patients, it was like a supreme self-disclosure – they saw that I am human, too. I do not simply exist in the shared space of the office, floating in suspension until their next session. I too am made of flesh and blood; I live in a house with a family, with animals, with neighbors and street noises and technological glitches. I also did not want to get sick from this virus. I was as disturbed by the current state of the world as they were; I was as affected by political upheaval, by uncertainty, by strangely shifting tides and by the fear that the whole world is in peril. Same as them.

As I grew accustomed to Zoom, I began to discern the more subtle differences of working remotely, in separate physical spaces. When we see patients in our offices, we unconsciously gather bits of information from all our senses. Our attention roams and all our wits are engaged. We perceive the bodily presence of our patients in various ways – the whiff of perfume, the smell of tawny leather, the spicy scent of a hastily eaten burrito – or the sound of their rushing footsteps coming down the hall, the rustle of their down jacket, the pinging of their phone – or the sensation of their physical presence – their girth, their shuffle, the particular slope of their shoulders or their habit of twirling their hair into a thick unruly top bun.

By now, we are likely all familiar with staring at our patients through the screen, as opposed to sitting with them. The Zoom camera strangely magnifies certain things that normally fade into the background when we are sitting together, in person, with our patients. On Zoom, our eyes are fixed, peering at the screen, overcompensating with our gaze for the missing data. Like our patients, we are strained by the loneliness of our isolation from others. Our chairs at home may be less comfortable than in our offices, the animals we live with may meander in and out of the session, even the sight of dirty dishes from our quickly downed breakfast or a sandwich, waiting for a lunch break, beckoning to us, placed carefully out of the camera's view – the details that surround us are reminders of being here, not there – in our literal houses, not in our offices.

Sometimes, in a Zoom session with a patient, I find myself focusing so intently that without noticing I lean closer and closer to the screen, as if I could slip through to the other side and be present with my patient, face to face, metabolizing all that we've discussed. My eyes fix on the screen, and I forget, momentarily, that I am actually in a room in my house, by myself. I am listening for all that I am worth.

And I sometimes remember that just as their faces are magnified on my screen, so is mine. I see my patients peer at me, reading my expressions up close. Such moments sometimes feel strangely intimate, as though something is revealed through the screen that might be missed in the office, where close scrutiny isn't always possible. It is as if all is exposed, my face revealing itself in magnification. At the beginning of the pandemic, I wondered, as I'm sure we all did, what would our work look like? Was it really sustainable to work via technology, never able to be together? Was there enough glue to hold the therapeutic action, to sustain the work and keep it alive?

When the call with a patient is over, the exit from this liminal space felt abrupt – one click and we're gone, barely take a beat before clicking on the next. We lost the in-between spaces – the crossings over the threshold, the openings and closings of the door, the walk down the hall from office to waiting room and back again at the end.

Working remotely, we lost the transitional moments that allow us to situate ourselves in the analytic frame – the very particular threshold-crossing in and out of the oasis of safety that our offices represent. Losing this passage made these few minutes remarkable in their absence – minutes that on ordinary days we barely take note of, so busy are we with what just happened and what is about to come – minutes we might spend checking our phones, or glancing out the window, fixing our hair, sipping tea, taking a breath between the end of one hour and the beginning of the next. Working on Zoom, I am jarred by the abrupt endings and beginnings, by the sense of popping in and out like the parody of a thought bubble. Time seems to warp and weave of its own accord, untethered by the usual landmarks. It drags, it flies, it is interrupted, it resumes, as jerky as an overly cautious driver shifting gears and pumping the brakes at the same time. In reality, there is no time between hours, one hour simply slides into the next, it is our rituals that give each hour its own miniature frame, creating the sensation that something has ended, something about to begin. I try to remember, had I ever really noticed those minutes, valued them, held them close in the palm of my hand? Had I ever known how quickly they could slip through my fingers?

There are moments where the particular intensity of Zoom may unexpectedly deepen the treatment. Once, a patient who went into foster care as a young boy pulled up a childhood photo and shared his screen with me.

Together, we bore witness to a small child, dressed for church in a button-down blouse with a little bowtie around his neck, long trousers tied with a belt and polished black lace-up shoes. His expression was inscrutable, face scrunched up in the hot sunlight, a serious look on his face. He stared straight into the camera. At some distance, a young woman stood apart from him, gazing into the distance – his birth mother, who disappeared and abandoned him just two weeks after the photo was taken. Three young other boys in the photo brandished sticks in their hands, raising their arms in the air, in mussed shirts and muddied pants, out of breath, hair askew, mouths wide open as if you could practically hear their shouts. The photo was a poignant testimony to the isolation and strain of a small boy keeping a secret so hefty he could not whisper it even to himself. Each from our own laptop in our own room, physically apart yet bound together by the intimacy of this moment, we peered together at the photo which filled up the screen. My patient began to weep. "No one has ever looked at this with me", he told me, "I've never shown it to anyone". In this moment, it was as if the ghost boy in the photo came alive in the virtual space that spanned the physical distance between us, creating simultaneously the needed space and the affective connection that made it possible to arc backwards in time and cradle his childhood pain.

Another such moment occurred in a session with an eight-year old patient I'll call Emily. She often liked to have her mother join the session at the beginning, as she said, "to get her started". This time, testing her readiness for a bit more autonomy, she asked her mother to join the session from another room. So, there we were in our Hollywood squares: mother on her phone on the third floor of their house, child on her iPad in the playroom, and me on the opposite side of my screen. Haltingly, Emily told me of a worry she had about picking the skin around her toenails, where callouses had formed from her soccer cleats. She did this at night, before going to sleep, but she worried that it would hurt her feet, and she didn't think it was right for her to do it.

Puzzled, I queried, "Right? How so?" Emily looked away, and her mother stepped in, gently encouraging her to tell me about "the other thing". Emily froze. She looked small and alone in her Zoom box. I suggested that maybe it would be easier for her to tell me if she were together in the same room as her mom. Immediately, she nodded. Her screen disappeared, and minutes later she popped into her mother's frame and jumped up on the bed. Curling up under her mother's solid embrace, she whispered that she was worried about touching her body at night, because she thought this was a very bad thing to do, not right at all. I asked her, "Why might you have the idea that it's a bad thing for you to do?" Nestling her head beneath her mother's encircling arm, Emily revealed that when she was in preschool, she'd been sharply reprimanded by a teacher during naptime for doing just that. "She shouted at me, using my whole name!" she burst out, and tears flowed down her cheeks.

While her mother embraced her, I marveled at the intimacy of the three of us, coming together via Zoom, at the vital experience of this young child grappling bravely with the intensity of her feelings and the power of her body, helping her recognize the risk of holding onto a secret filled with pain and shame – listening to her mother's assurances that her body was hers to explore and experiment with, that human biology contains wonder, and that such feelings need not be kept hidden as shameful secrets.

These moments revealed to me both what is possible via Zoom, and simultaneously what cannot be attained in a virtual world. My older patient revealed a silent truth about a painful past that he could not put into words. Later, he told me that he remembered what that day felt like, keeping himself away from the rollicking games of his friends, and felt the old tightening in his core of his childhood fear.

Emily shared something she may have felt too shy or ashamed to tell me had we been together in my office. Yet at the same time, it seemed impossible to put words to her bodily sensations and confusing emotions without the comfort and safety of her mother's embrace. What is her experience of her own physicality, I wondered, when she cannot inhabit the physical world in all of its familiar contours – separated from friends, teachers, and relatives, cut off from the sensory feedback we get from touch? It was only when she felt held securely in her mother's arms that she could unburden herself of her secret shame and the fears that came with it.

And so, while Zoom allows for the illusion of being together, we all hungered for the physicality of the ordinary world. We longed for the casual gestures of holding hands, linking arms, hugging one another in greeting and farewell. We grew weary of being disembodied heads and shoulders bobbing in our boxes and peering out through our screens.

"I miss the bodies!" 29-year-old Martha said to me. "I want to feel the heat, the crush! I want to go to a club and dance and feel the sweat of other people's bodies. I don't even like clubs – but I want all the touch!"

The technology allows us to continue our work with our patients, true, but no one could argue that it's the same. My patients often complain of being weary of Zoom – not just the effort of looking at the screen, but also of the strange state of together-yet-apart that we all feel to some degree. I have a few patients who prefer to not use Zoom at all. With some of them, I have developed a ritual of walking during sessions, albeit separately, and talking – each of us donning jackets, boots and earphones, leaving our houses at the exact same moment and talking together as we walk, as though being situated in the physical world allows them to feel once again the solidity of our connection. With one young patient, Louie, this ritual emerged because he could not bear the experience of Zoom for our sessions, and found himself growing sadder and sadder, cutting the sessions short. Then we began to walk. Throughout summer, fall and winter, Louie would call at his appointed hour, and we would each set out, commenting from time to time on what we were seeing. "Hold on a sec, I have to cross the street", he'd tell me. "Oh my gosh, there is the cutest dog over there! Hiya, pup!" On these walks, I would pass by the same particularly broad tree, noticing its transformation from a rich, full green canopy of leaves, to a red-gold crown, to bare branches crackling in the wind.

I realized that the walks had become important to me too – a way of marking time – and that Louie had become once again intensely engaged in our work together.

From time to time in Zoom sessions, I found myself acutely aware of the screen – whether I noticed the contours of the laptop or glimpsed my image in the tiny box at the top of the screen, my face now distorted and bug-eyed from leaning too close to the camera, or momentarily startled by a pop-up alert because I'd forgotten to shut down my notifications. This in-between space I'd been inhabiting with the patient, a kind of half-real, half-imagined space, an illusory technicolor intimacy, is fragile and prone to shatter.

Working this way requires a certain energy expended in denial (of our separation) and a suspension of disbelief (that we are, in fact, virtually together). We must be willing to sign on, at least in part, to the illusion that we are still together – a kind of as-if experience of togetherness. Twenty-year-old Hallie told me, "Technology is like an almost-replacement, we can feel almost the same as being together, but it's not, we're really not together, it's not a real replacement. Once during the pandemic, I snuck out, I went to my friend's house, I felt guilty. But then the five of us just hung out and smoked pot, it felt so real, so normal! We stayed up till 4 in the morning – we literally had no idea what time it was, because time doesn't mean anything anymore to any of us. But it felt so good! I didn't want it to end". This paradox allows a glimpse of both the essence of humanity – the need to be alive amongst other humans – and the need to build resilience, sustain our momentum, survive our isolation.

Today, some patients still extol the virtues of meeting on-line, saving the time it takes to get to the office, being able to meet comfortably at home, in their pajamas even, not having to take time off work, or even being able to share with me their pets who wander in and out of the room, or photos they put up on the screen, or even the occasional sighting of a family member ducking into the room. But for others, this period of time led to a sense of disconnection, despair and unbearable loneliness.

What of our younger patients, whether children, adolescents or young adults, for whom the real possibility of mortality can prematurely shatter the optimistic future they had begun to envision? Jack, a 24-year-old patient, said to me, "I was so ready and excited, leaving school – it's like it's all been taken away. Time is flying but I'm not making any memories, in my mind I'm just pushing to keep going until I can see the thing I want to do. I just have to get through, but how long until COVID breaks? My dreams for the future are bleeding out. What's my life now? Stalled, surreal and weird". I nod. I see that Jack's cat has wandered into his room and jumped on the back of the couch. It crawls onto his shoulder, curling its tail around Jack's head and looking straight at me. Jack reaches his arm toward the cat and scratches its neck. His features soften, and I see the cat, too, close its eyes in feline bliss.

Jack lifts the cat onto his lap and shakes his head. "I'm just waiting to resume", he goes on. "I'm putting Band-Aids on my desires. There's something so crazy about how I've used time. I found out how to cope when I feel empty. I'm unfulfilled by my relationships, I can't operate how I normally would. My sense of agency is extinct. I feel clueless, swimming in a world where I can't breathe".

He pauses for a moment, thinking. "Maybe that's why I play video games the way I do – they are moral and uncompromised, non-negotiable. It's the most relaxing part of my day – I start, I finish, it grabs my attention completely. Normally, I feel I can grab onto my whole life fully, like I have control, but now I have no control. Now I'm scared I don't know what's real, what's profound – I'm just pushing everything away". How, I think, can he find a safe perch, a place for reflection, a way to look back at all of this, when it is all still happening?

While for younger patients, the pandemic and the ensuing isolation thrust mortality into premature awareness, older patients experienced the anguish of lost time, knowing it can no longer be salvaged. Lucille, a woman in her seventies whose husband died during the pandemic, remarked to me, "I feel like I'm in a snow globe that's been turned upside down. For the first time in my life, I feel that there are no anchors to this world. Nothing seems real, anything is possible. When's the last time I had a full belly laugh? Who am I going to laugh with now? I am being robbed of my time on this earth and there is nothing I can do to stop it".

Indeed, like a snow globe, while we have been lying fallow, confined, constrained, our contact with others restricted, the world around us has been turned upside down, the debris that has gathered over years has been disturbed, and we have all been shaken out of complacency. How, I wonder, will we find our way back to ourselves? We have seen our patients respond in a multitude of ways to having lost the experience of human contact, of being out in the world, amongst others. There is nowhere to turn to refresh. And yet, for some, living in solitude has loosened old restraints and constraints – it has opened internal spaces, where we can no longer turn our eyes away from the problems that are embedded *within us*.

This time has brought the awakening of the Black Lives Matter movement, and the stark dangers that make our society vulnerable to fracture. This period of COVID, and the devastation it has wrought, knows no bounds – it afflicts the poor and the wealthy, the vulnerable and the healthy. But its sweep across the nation has also revealed the vast chasms that exist among us, separating race, class, caste and culture. It has revealed the rifts and has challenged us to look deeply into what has been ruined and tarnished in our world. While the world has been tilted on its axis, the imbalances amongst us have reached a precarious tipping point. They call for recognition and reconciliation. The painful realities of our existing system, one that has inherently supported dangerous and often fatal inequities in race and caste, in economics and healthcare, in education and aging, have been laid bare in ways we cannot ignore.

As psychoanalysts, it is also our time to face the facts that have been laid bare within our own community. In our period of confinement, we have, by necessity, tested the walls of our therapeutic frame. We have nearly all turned to technology where once we would have eschewed such ruptures to the rhythm of our work. We have seen our patients from within our homes, viewed the interior spaces within which our patients reside – before COVID, would we have ever shared with our colleagues that we are seeing our patients sitting in their cars, or closeted in their pantries, or, for some, even huddled under the covers?

Tested by the need to persevere with our work in ways we may never have conceived, the psychoanalytic frame endures, bent but not broken, as we strive to gain flexibility, wisdom, resilience and elasticity. Who will we be when we emerge?

Post-Script

I wrote this essay during the height of the pandemic, with no certainty about what was to come – when would the COVID lockdown be over, and what would things look like in the aftermath.

We have all been through this together, and have emerged into a world far noisier, messier and more chaotic than the one we recall. And still, we can't know what lies ahead of us in the future.

In retrospect, getting the first COVID vaccine was destined to become one of those moments – *where were you when Kennedy was shot? When 9/11 happened? When you got your first COVID vaccine?* I remember crying tears I didn't expect – as if I didn't fully know how scared, and weird, and uncertain, and disturbed I'd been feeling during those long months of isolation.

Sometimes I imagine that the best view we will have of the COVID era will be telescoped back from the future, with a wide enough angle to capture all of the turmoil beneath the surface, like the subtle shifting of tectonic plates or the crashing of waves against a ragged shoreline.

As psychoanalysts, we continue to ponder what happened during those years, What were the effects of our profession shifting, as if in unison, to virtual psychoanalysis? During the pandemic, it was our primary source of connectedness, and as such we drank it thirstily, relieved to be able to meet with our patients, to try to weave together as best we could the threads of the analyses we were engaged with. Nearly all of us experienced a variety of strategies to persevere. Fearful for our patients, concerned about their experiences, concerned about our own, we gradually found a way forward, consulting one another often and marveling at how different things had become.

As the world opened up once again, we wondered how to make meaning of what had taken place during the time of COVID. Some patients couldn't wait to return to the office in person, often tearful and overwhelmed in the initial in-person sessions. Others opted to continue via Zoom, having discovered something they wanted to hold onto – whether a new-found intimacy on the screen, or a literal improvement (e.g., a patient of mine who suffered hearing loss discovered she could hear much better on Zoom), or others simply reclaiming the time it took them to commute to our offices. Similarly, some of my own colleagues now meet virtually only reluctantly, while others have given up their offices entirely and work exclusively online. So, what have we learned?

It is true that not being together in the same space felt very different. We found we relied less on the subtle physical cues we are accustomed to tuning into in person, and more on minute changes in facial expression, speech tempo, disruptions in associations and visual cues. There may be differences in how we begin, how we end, how able we are to manage the in-between spaces.

But still, our patients rely on the steady heartbeat of the treatment that makes psychoanalytic work possible. Rather than focusing on what we have gleaned about the benefits and drawbacks of working virtually, perhaps the more vital question is, what has zoom work revealed to us about the practice of psychoanalysis itself? Virtual psychoanalysis has exposed the raw nerve of the analytic encounter, stripping away the familiar to reveal what is essential, what is transformational. Our virtual consulting rooms have spotlighted the resilience and elasticity of the analytic endeavor.

The analyst's listening presence may take on new dimensions when filtered through technology.[1] Patients may experience the analyst's presence more intensely, as if the focused gaze peering through the screen amplifies a sense of emotional connectedness. We notice the impact of what we reveal and what we conceal on screen – even the digital glitches we encounter carry the echoes of our patients' and our own, inarticulable fears and desires: *Are you still there? Can you hear me? My connection is weak. You are frozen.* This heightened listening reveals the myriad ways in which analytic work picks up the even faintest signals of the unconscious, regardless of the medium.

The analytic relationship – one which we always assumed would require physical presence –has proven to be a robust psychic construct. In a unique paradox, the screen simultaneously separates and connects, creating a particular form of intimacy. The zoom environment – whether visible or blurred in the background, whether in the home, car or hiding in the bathroom so as not to be overheard, the ways that patient and analyst settle into the session on screen, or how they handle inevitable disturbances – all have become rich text for analysis.

Perhaps most profoundly, virtual analysis has reinforced that insight and change do not stem from the frame created within the consulting room itself, but from the quality of the space created between analyst and patient, as defined by analytic listening, and the emergence of shared meanings, unexpected moments of humor or surprise, and uncanny revelations. Insights are discovered, dreams are unpacked, the transference/countertransference theater plays out on our screens. The unconscious still makes itself known.

The core of psychoanalytic work – the capacity to plumb the depths of the unconscious, to hold and transform emotional experiences, and to foster genuine self-discovery – is not bound by physical constraints. Instead, it adapts in the face of changing circumstances and continuously forges new pathways for analytic work to unfold.

This was brought home to me when a patient recently flew into town to have our termination in person. He had moved away during the pandemic and we had continued our work online.

We agreed that he would stay for one week and we would meet every day that week. Seeing me in person felt deeply important to him. He couldn't imagine saying goodbye on Zoom. "What would we do?" he wondered aloud. "I can't imagine ending years of working together with just one click and you're gone".

At the beginning of the in-person termination week, he felt exuberant, sensing that he had been able to knit himself together during the analysis and felt equipped for whatever might fall in his path. He expressed grief at ending the work and gratitude for what we had accomplished. On the last day, he announced as he came into the office that his doctor had just called him with some worrisome lab results. "I'm going in for a CAT scan when I get back", he said. "Maybe we didn't pick the best week to terminate after all". Having lost both of his parents quite young, he felt frightened, discouraged and deflated. We talked about his fears that all the gains he'd felt he'd made might vanish in a flash, slip through his fingers and disappear. We agreed that he could contact me if he felt it would be helpful. A tear slipped down his face.

In the last ten minutes of the hour, he fixed his gaze on the clock, watching each minute tick by. He rested quietly in the chair, commenting on how familiar it felt, how securely it held his girth, how the leather felt smooth and worn. When the ten minutes elapsed, he looked over at me.

"I thought I would want to hug you", he said, "but I find that I don't need that. I don't really want it. You have held me and I feel that". At the threshold, he turned to me and reached out his arms toward me, palms outstretched. It was as if the gesture contained all of the spaces between us – the distance from my chair to where he stood at the door, the hug he longed for and the physical separation between us, the virtual space of our time meeting through the Zoom screen, all the liminal spaces where the analysis unfolded over the years. For a moment, he held me in his gaze, then smiled a bit.

"Here you are", he said, bringing his hands together at his heart. "Here I go". Then he crossed over the threshold, leaving the door ajar.

Note

1 Adelman, A. (2021). Through the looking glass: Holding the analytic frame on zoom. *American Imago, 78*(3), 491–501. © 2021 Johns Hopkins University Press. Reprinted with permission of Johns Hopkins University Press.

9 Caught in the Crossfire

Political Intersections, Collisions, and Confrontations[1]

Karen E. Starr

Recent political events in our own country and around the world are reverberating loudly in the consulting room. In the course of my clinical work, I am daily reminded, with an intensity I have not heretofore experienced, that the political is personal and the personal, political. As current events ignite new anxieties and enflame old ones, power dynamics that rear their ugly heads in the political sphere often resonate with those we have experienced in our personal lives. Whether we are patients or analysts, we are all in the same boat, embedded in the larger social and political forces of the world we live in. Despite our relative position of authority within the psychoanalytic dyad, our role as analyst does not shield us from feelings of powerlessness in the face of a national and global catastrophe that continues to unfold on a daily basis.

One of my patients, an artist who identifies as lesbian, grew up having to negotiate the vagaries of a tyrannical and narcissistic father, the CEO of a large corporation, who was openly critical of her sexual identity and dismissive of her choice of profession. The election of Donald Trump as president both reactivated and amplified her childhood fear that she lived at the mercy of a man who could very well crush her or pull the rug out from under her financially if she made the wrong move. In reference to the flurry of executive orders coming out of the White House, she recently told me, "I wake up every morning to the harsh reality that what I have always dreaded could happen, but told myself would never happen, is actually happening right now".

Little did she know that with these words, she was giving voice to exactly what I was feeling. Like our patients, we analysts are not immune to the harsh realities of current events, or to the reverberations of past trauma stimulated by these events, whether it be in our individual, family, or cultural histories, or in echoes of experience that have been passed down to us through the generations.

I'm somewhat embarrassed to say that, prior to the 2016 election, I would have unselfconsciously described myself as "not a political person". I have since come to realize that the phrase "not a political person" is an impossibility. As individuals born into a particular time, place, and social surround, according to Althusser (1970), we are "always-already interpellated by ideology as subjects" (p. 119). Advocating for a psychoanalysis that incorporates the

DOI: 10.4324/9781003584803-13

social, psychoanalyst Nancy Hollander (2017) articulated the ways in which symbolic structures of power and authority may be internalized by the individual as aspects of personal identity. Awoken from its slumber by a visceral state of alarm, my political self has been newly activated by the election of Donald Trump as 45th President of the United States.

Echoes of Experience

Until then, I had always felt myself to be on the periphery, observing politics from the sidelines. Having been born at the very tail end of the baby boom, a child of the 60s who was just a child in the 60s, I papered the walls of my bedroom with psychedelic flowers and practiced writing my name in bubble letters while the news on TV showed soldiers being carried out of Vietnam in body bags. My brother, who was 12 years older than me, was of draft-eligible age. His college cancelled classes because of student "sit-ins". Talk of deferment and lottery numbers anxiously swirled around the dinner table. My brother's friends joked about becoming rabbis to avoid the draft and potentially Vietnam, while my brother's solution was to preemptively enlist in the National Guard. He came home from his five months of basic training startlingly skinny and with his head shaved smooth as an almond, announcing his arrival by waking me up with an early morning reveille – clanging a metal spoon against a pot, so I would get a taste of what military life was like. I marveled at the medal he earned for marksmanship; it depicted two rifles, crossed, with a rainbow of stars. I could not imagine my brother holding a rifle, let alone knowing how to shoot it. Two of his peers had been killed by "friendly fire" during practice exercises; my 9-year-old self could not get her head around this paradoxical phrase. Fortunately, my brother completed his service without incident. It was only much later as an adult that I realized the shootings of the college students at Kent State had been at the hands of the National Guard (Kifner, 1970, May 5).

Although I observed the political upheaval of the 60s from the outside looking in, my parents' immigrant experience was deeply embedded in my psyche. My parents were refugees from the Holocaust who had known each other in Vienna but had each fled separately after the Nazi invasion. The dangerous world they had inhabited and only narrowly escaped was visible in the blue numbers tattooed on the arms of many of the adults in my parents' circle; its echoes reverberated in the cadence of their accented speech. The neighborhood where I grew up, in the Inwood section of Manhattan, was populated with refugees from Europe. While I played with my friends in the Fort Tryon Park playground, our mothers sat on the bench talking, their voices a symphony of Hungarian, Polish, Czech, and German. Our parents' pasts were the background music of our childhoods.

In Maus (1986), his graphic novel of the Holocaust, Art Spiegelman wrote, "My father bleeds history". My father spread it on pumpernickel toast with butter and garlic and fed it to me for breakfast. As he cut my sandwiches into hearts and my radishes into roses, he recounted over and over, and over again, the stories of the life he had lived before I was born. Sitting across from my father at the kitchen table, I listened to his stories, as if, by listening hard enough, I could take his pain from him. I felt my father's fright when he was told by his employer that the Gestapo were coming for him; his anger that life as he knew it was falling apart; his desperation to find refuge for himself and his infant daughter, my half-sister. I felt his humiliation when, having been betrayed by his beloved Vienna, he was faced with anti-Semitism even in America, the country that had given him refuge but was loathe to give a job to an immigrant Jew. "You can wipe your ass with your diploma", said the Southern textile mill owner to my father in response to his presenting his credentials, a degree in chemistry from the University of Vienna.

My father's fear that catastrophe could strike again, even in America, the land that had tolerated but not welcomed him, remained unspoken, but in the air. Today, news of a Muslim ban, immigration roundups, and white nationalists marching with torches sends my father's fear coursing through my body, mingled with my own. I am aware that while the specifics of the designation "shithole countries" (Dawsey, 2018, January 12) might change in any given era, the sentiment behind these vulgar words remains chillingly the same. I don't just "know" this, I feel it in my bones.

My mother was 21 when she fled the Nazis by embarking on a boat to what was then British Mandated Palestine, with the hopeful goal of reuniting with and eventually marrying my father in America. It was only by snooping through the papers my father kept in his beautifully polished maple wood box when I was 15 that I discovered the document certifying my mother's divorce from a man whose name I did not recognize. It was then I learned that the passengers on that boat, many of them strangers, had married one another for the purpose of obtaining a place on the ship. In the British quota system, a married couple counted as only one person. My mother spent four years on kibbutz and then another four years, penniless and starving, in Havana, Cuba, repeatedly denied entry to the United States. The U.S. government, at war with Austria, the country that exterminated the family she left behind, had classified her as an "enemy alien".

"Enemy alien". My father bitterly repeated these words to me, cursing the U.S. immigration system for its perverse cruelty and berating himself for not knowing better how to navigate it. I was named Karen for the Jewish girl in the novel *Exodus* (Uris, 1958) whose father sent her out of Nazi Germany to safety while he stayed behind and perished. The actual ship, the *Exodus 1947,* had in real life become a symbol of illegal immigration. Embarking from Europe to British Mandated Palestine, the *Exodus* was filled with refugees from the Holocaust, many of whom did not have legal immigration certificates. To set an example, the British stopped the *Exodus* and refused it entry, sending it and its passengers back to Germany, where they were forced off the ship and sent to detention camps. Such was the legacy of immigration into which I was born.

The Past as Prelude to the Present

Anticipating a historic victory by the first-ever woman candidate for President of the United States, the Democratic nominee, Secretary of State and former New York Senator Hillary Clinton, my then 23-year-old twin daughters and I spent the evening of Election Day, November 8, 2016, excitedly texting back and forth as we watched the news. Imagine, a female President, in our lifetime! By 10 p.m., our excitement turned to dread as the voting data increasingly pointed to a Donald Trump victory. "President Trump" read the news headline on my phone when I woke up at 2 a.m. It was inconceivable, but true. I was devastated. On my way to work the day after, there was a strange hush among my fellow commuters. It felt eerily like the quiet pall that had enveloped the city after 9/11, as if New York City was once again engaged in collective mourning.

The sense of foreboding I felt the day after Election Day was indeed a harbinger of nightmarish events yet to come. Xenophobic, misogynistic, and nationalist election rhetoric has now come to life in the form of racist, anti-immigrant, anti-woman, and anti-LGBTQ policies emanating from the White House, facilitated by a complicit Congress. I cannot help but hear echoes of 1930s Germany in the thinly veiled racist pronouncements of the President and his government appointees. I recognize, as if remembering, the perverse cruelty of Border Patrol agents destroying bottles of water left by humanitarian groups for migrants crossing the Arizona desert (Wang, 2018, January 24); and of Immigration and Customs Enforcement (ICE) agents separating hundreds of asylum seekers from their children (Kennedy, 2018, March 9). It all feels eerily familiar, as if the ghosts of the past are haunting me in the present. As I watch these events unfold, I realize that I am bearing witness to them in the here-and-now through the telescopic lens (Faimberg, 2005) of my parents' past. Keenly attuned to the tremors of history whose rumblings, to my ear, are audible in the current political climate, I am alarmed, perhaps in a way that others with a different history might not be. However, from conversations with colleagues, and from presenting this paper at psychoanalytic conferences and other professional venues, I know that many of us carry with us our own unique family histories of trauma and immigration, as well as our own relationship to politics and political action. Many of us are alarmed. Awareness and acknowledgment of our own location in history and politics is essential if we are to be aware of and address historical trauma and the political environment in which we live.

Over this past year and a half, in sitting with my patients, I have had the uncanny experience of being caught in the crossfire of current events and transgenerational trauma, of competing subjectivities and conflicting political views. I found myself asking myself these questions: As analysts, how do we attend to and empathize with our patients' experience, including their political views, when they conflict with ours? How do we help our patients give voice to their values and beliefs while helping them see other perspectives?

What happens when political fervor eclipses human compassion? Given our position of authority within the psychoanalytic dyad, is it our responsibility to bracket our subjective experience and political beliefs in order to allow our patients' voices to emerge, or is it in fact our responsibility to speak up to give voice to that which is not being said? Given our position of influence, what do we have to teach our patients about the value of political engagement, and, if we allow ourselves to be influenced, what might we learn from them?

It is my hope these questions can serve as a starting point for a conversation among us about how to navigate the turbulent waters of our current political situation without sinking the boat of our analytic responsibility. For now, I offer two brief case vignettes. In the first, I was dismayed to encounter my non-political self in my patient, Theresa. This encounter led me to question whether my analytic responsibility necessitated educating my patient about politics, or whether it required me to exclusively stay close to her experience. In the second, while feeling uncertain about my own ability to have an impact, either clinically or politically, I found inspiration in my patient, Sam. Inviting Sam to be my teacher helped each of us, in our own way, access a sense of agency in the face of forces we experienced as beyond our control.

Radical Muslim Extremists

Theresa, age 24, came to see me, she said, because she was experiencing significant anxiety that she attributed to her stressful new job. She had been anxious for as long as she could remember, but it had gotten to a point where her mother, with whom she was very close, told her she needed to talk to someone. Theresa lived at home with her parents and brother, who were ardent Trump supporters and Fox News viewers. The discussions in Theresa's house were often heated and often centered on politics. Her father and brother dominated the conversation. Theresa described her father as volatile and moody, and her brother as stubborn and loud. She felt sorry for her mother, who had to tiptoe around her father's moods, but she was also angry with her for not standing up to him. Theresa felt that all the men in her family, including her grandfathers, bullied the women.

It soon became clear that, while Theresa's new job was indeed stressful, her intense anxiety stemmed from a different source. She had been keeping a secret from her parents, and the secrecy was tearing her apart. Unbeknownst to her parents, at least so Theresa believed, she was involved in a clandestine relationship with her former high school sweetheart. They had broken up years ago, when they were teenagers, because her parents disapproved of him. But Theresa came to admit to herself – and to me – that he was her first and only love. Theresa's young man was handsome and sweet, and while the men in her family and the other men she had dated all talked "at" her, he listened. He was an accountant, just like her dad.

The problem? Theresa's boyfriend, Bashir, was Muslim. His parents immigrated to the United States from Iran when he was a child. Theresa seemed vaguely aware that her parents' political views colored their attitude toward Bashir. Yet she was unable to connect the dots between her parents' prejudice, the surrounding political rhetoric, and her personal situation. When I inquired specifically about her own political views, Theresa responded with a giggle, "I'm not a political person". She told me she's not sure she will vote, but if she does, she will most probably vote for Trump, because that's what her family will do. Of course, they all hate "Hillary". Internally, I winced. I said something gentle about the irony of that, given her current dilemma, but it went over her head. Theresa's lack of political consciousness seemed almost deliberate; I suspected it was her way of protecting herself from venturing too far from her family.

Theresa was torn. She loved her parents and did not want to be disloyal, but she knew Bashir was the love of her life, and she did not want to give him up. She wanted to tell her parents, but she was afraid they would disown her. The thought of losing him or losing them tied her in knots. Not being truthful, especially with her mother, was torture. Theresa suspected that her mother suspected. She knew her so well, how could she not know? For several months, Theresa and I worked together on the possibility of her telling her parents, or at least, at first, her mother. One morning, on the day of her scheduled session, Theresa left me a voice mail. "Heads up", said Theresa's voice on the recording. "I told my mother. She's coming to my session". I braced myself.

All day, I was on edge. I spent the day thinking about my experience as a young adult, when, during a college semester abroad in Israel, I had fallen in love with a handsome Israeli paratrooper. His parents, who were from Iraq, warmly welcomed me with open arms, treating me like family. They were my home away from home. They knew no English, only Hebrew and Arabic, and so we communicated in a combination of both. When my mother came to visit, they treated her like an honored guest, preparing a feast for her of Iraqi delicacies. It made her sick to her stomach, literally and figuratively. "Primitive", she called them. It made no difference to her that they were Jews who had fled religious persecution in Iraq. She threatened to stop paying my college tuition if I continued to see him and eventually followed through on her threat.

Back in my office, Theresa's mother, Connie, sat on the couch at the edge of her seat, while Theresa huddled in the opposite corner, arms crossed, a sullen expression on her face. "I want to talk", said Connie. "Please let me talk. I have a lot I want to get off my chest". I invited her to speak. "Radical Muslim extremists", she announced, staring at me intently, waiting for my reaction, as if preparing for battle. I stayed quiet. "Radical Muslim extremists are a threat to our safety and to this country". Her tone was urgent. "Look at the bombings in Paris. What happened there could happen here. You must agree with me that the situation is very frightening. The Obama administration has been completely ineffective; it has done nothing to protect us".

Instinctively, I held up my hand to stop her. I knew no good could come from going down that road. "Of course, the bombings were terrible and frightening. But my politics are very different from yours", I said. "Why don't we leave politics aside for now and focus on your concerns about Theresa". Oddly, Connie appeared relieved. She seemed to appreciate my directness. She sat back on the couch.

"Do you believe Bashir is a radical Muslim extremist?" I asked. Connie was silent for a few moments. "No", she said softly, "I don't. I think he's a nice boy. I just worry that there's so much hatred of Muslims in this country. I know how people talk about Muslims. I don't want Theresa to be subjected to that". She turned to her daughter, "I'm afraid of how Muslim men treat their women. I don't want you to be in an oppressive relationship. I don't want that for you. How does he treat you? Does he let you talk?"

"Yes, Mom", Theresa said. She was crying. "He lets me talk. He is the only man I have ever met who lets me talk".

Humanizing the "Other"

Sam, a doctoral candidate in History, was suffering from a severe depressive episode, precipitated by his fiancée suddenly, without warning, leaving him for another man. Her betrayal was a bombshell, shattering his life as he knew it, obliterating everything he thought he could take for granted. Together, we struggled to make sense of her motives, and of how Sam had been so blindsided. He had not seen it coming. Or was there something coming he had not wanted to see? To cast the shadow of his fiancée's betrayal retrospectively over their five-year relationship was too much for Sam to bear. To preserve her goodness and the goodness of the life they shared together, Sam blamed only himself. His anger turned inward, his self-recrimination was relentless, fueling his pervasive feelings of hopelessness and despair, reinforcing his sense of himself as worthless and innately unlovable. His sentences trailed off, unfinished, as if it was useless for him even to try to speak his thoughts aloud. I struggled to find a way in, to locate any aspect of Sam's identity that could anchor him to a sense of his own goodness and his own agency. Nothing I said seemed to penetrate his self-defeating narrative. His world was in ruins, and all he could do was sift through the ashes.

In an uncanny parallel of art imitating life, Sam's dissertation was about the terror attacks of 9/11, attempting to make sense of its causes and repercussions. Sam's research examined the historical and political factors leading up to this tragic event, including the pattern of U.S. intervention in the Middle East; as well as how the resulting U.S. military response, the war on Iraq, contributed to the formation of ISIS, the radical extremist Islamic State. While talking about the breakup only made Sam feel worse, talking with me about his dissertation seemed to give him some relief. He was soft-spoken and thoughtful, even articulate. I discovered, with some surprise, that Sam was an excellent teacher. I became his interested student.

I invited Sam to teach me about Middle Eastern history, about Islam, and about political theory. We talked about the devastation of 9/11; about how, in the aftermath, the city seemed to come together for a little while, and how comforting that was. I shared with him that I was in the World Trade Center bombing in 1993–in retrospect, a precursor to 9/11. Pregnant with twins, I ran down 79 flights of stairs, my face black with smoke. It was snowing outside. As first responders boarded me in an ambulance, a stranger, a statuesque Black woman, gave me her coat. Her coat, bright red and voluminous, enveloped me with the warmth of her kindness. I have never forgotten it.

The Paris bombings (Nossiter & Gladstone, 2015, November 13) pulled Sam out of his depressive spiral of poring through his past to sift for clues and thrust him sharply into the present. Sam was alarmed by the attacks, but he was even more concerned about the impact on his students at the city college where he taught, many of whom were Muslim. Several had confided in him that they had already been targets of harassment, stirred up by the anti-Muslim 2016 election rhetoric. As a teacher, Sam was worried about his students. As a historian, he was concerned that the American political discourse characterizing Islam as a radical extremist religion would further polarize East from West. The shocking result of the presidential election, and the ensuing executive orders issued by the White House compounded Sam's concerns. Several of his Muslim students were caught up in the travel ban, unable to return to the United States for the start of the spring semester (Thrush, 2017).

Sam was not sure how to address these recent events and the resulting political discussions in his classroom. Was it his responsibility to his class and to the college to remain politically neutral and adhere to his lesson plan? Or, to the contrary, was it his responsibility to educate his students – to apply the lessons of history to the present, and to teach them about the dangers of nationalism and xenophobia? If he chose the latter, how could he make the classroom feel like a safe place for everyone, including those with opposing political viewpoints? The analytic hour became a space for us both to think about these questions. As we considered Sam's options for individual intervention in the face of larger political forces that felt beyond our control, I privately reflected on mine. As he wondered what he could do, even in a small way, to have an impact, I wondered, what could I?

Sam decided to do a "teach-in". He suspended his planned curriculum, and for three consecutive classes, taught his students about Islam and Islamic history. At the conclusion of his teach-in, Sam felt he had made the right decision. He believed that, for the moment, he had succeeded in his goal of humanizing those who were being targeted as "other". He felt a little bit better about himself, a little less hopeless, having newly connected with a sense of himself as having an impact, while acting in accordance with his values.

Heartened by this first sign of life in Sam, I encouraged him to continue thinking about how he might put his values into practice through his teaching. Given his passion for political theory, might there be a way he could engage his students to think more critically? Might there be some way to make the lessons of history more relevant to his students' everyday lives, by focusing their attention on what was happening in the world at that very moment? Sam took on the challenge. He revamped his curriculum, introducing a discussion of current events into every class discussion of historical political movements. While he was open with his students about his own political stance, he took great care to make his classroom a safe container for multiple viewpoints and a space for respectful dialogue.

In inviting Sam to be my teacher, I had found a way in. Through his teaching, Sam was able to access a feeling of agency and aliveness that had otherwise eluded him. In turn, my work with Sam benefited me. Not only did it expand my intellectual horizons, but also in helping Sam put his values into practice, I realized that I was putting mine into practice as well. My one-on-one clinical work with Sam potentiated a small ripple of change that – who knows?–may lead to a larger one. I, too, felt a little bit better, a little less hopeless, in the face of larger political forces that were beyond my control. Drawing upon the Jewish mystical concept of *tikkun olam*, or repair of the world, a metaphor I have also found useful for conceptualizing the psychoanalytic endeavor (Starr, 2008), Samuels (2017) suggested that helping our clients be "citizen-therapists for the wider world" may be good for the analysts' soul (p. 687). While I am hesitant to apply this formulation too broadly, in the case of my work with Sam, I believe it to be true.

I'll conclude these reflections with the words of Abraham Lincoln, a quite different Republican president. In words that ring as true today as they did 150 years ago, Lincoln (1859) said, "From the first appearance of man upon the earth down to very recent time, the words "stranger" and "enemy" were quite or almost synonymous. Even yet, this has not totally disappeared. The man of the highest moral cultivation . . . likes him whom he does know much better than him whom he does not know. To correct the evils, great and small, which spring from want of sympathy and from positive enmity among strangers, as nations or as individuals, is one of the highest functions of civilization".

January 2025 Reflection: "It's déjà vu All Over Again" (Berra, 1961)

In a sadly ironic turn of events, I am writing this reflection on my original paper just a week after Donald's Trump's second inauguration, as the 47th President of the United States. The past few days have brought a brutal onslaught of executive orders designed to terrorize undocumented immigrants and their families and to dehumanize and disenfranchise other marginalized communities. In the intervening years between now and when I first presented my paper at the APsA National Meeting self-disclosure discussion group in New York in 2018, my patients and I, along with the rest of the world, have also endured the COVID-19 global pandemic. Our shared experience of the pandemic and of our country's virulently divisive politics has underscored just how difficult, if not impossible, it is to disentangle the social and the political from an understanding of the personal. This time around, the question of how our respective subject positions interact with our political environment to impact what happens in the consulting room, seems even more relevant and pressing than ever.

In the days following this second Trump inauguration, many of my patients are grappling yet again with the question of how to preserve their mental wellbeing without becoming flooded and overwhelmed by the news, while at the same time staying aware of and attuned to what is happening in the world. Truthfully, I am too. Our analytic discourse has been rife with existential themes: What can one do in response to evil? What does it mean to be complicit? If we are powerless to stop the onslaught, does that mean we can do nothing? If we don't do something, are we not bystanders? Several patients, some of whom are also descendants of Holocaust survivors, have alluded to the facing the dilemma of "ordinary" Germans during the Nazi's rise to power. These analogies are understandable and, in my view, not overstated.

Some of my patients are clinicians themselves, working in community clinics treating a largely immigrant population. Sam, the doctoral student in history I wrote about in my original paper, is one of them. Now a therapist, Sam is thinking deeply about how to put his values into action both in terms of his social activism and in the context of the therapeutic relationship. As he put it, treating a patient's anxiety as if it were a standalone symptom emerging from intrapsychic conflict without explicitly acknowledging the terrifying reality that the patient's undocumented family members are under threat of deportation, would be a form of therapeutic malpractice.

This time around feels like it will be worse than the last. But this time around I am not so politically naïve as to feel blindsided. A young patient of mine, a Holocaust and Genocide historian, said to me, "I grew up believing Martin Luther King Jr., that the arc of history 'bends toward justice'.[2] But as a historian, I know it's not true. History doesn't bend toward justice. Bad things happen and then they happen again".

Notes

1 A version of this chapter was presented at the Facing the Facts: Self Disclosure and the Analytic Relationship discussion group, APsA National Meeting, New York City, February 2018. This chapter is adapted from Starr, K. E. (2018). Caught in the crossfire: Political intersections, collisions, and confrontations. *Psychoanalysis, Self, and Context, 13*, 389–397, reprinted by permission of Informa UK Limited, trading as Taylor & Francis Group, www.tandfonline.com.

2 The actual quote is "We shall overcome because the arc of the moral universe is long, but it bends toward justice." From Martin Luther King, Jr.'s sermon at the Washington National Cathedral, March 31, 1968.

References

Althusser, L. (1970). Ideology and ideological state apparatus. In *Lenin and philosophy* (pp. 85–126). New York: Monthly Review Press.

Berra, Y. (1961). Retrieved January 25, 2025 from https://yogiberramuseum.org/about-yogi/yogisms/#:~:text=%E2%80%9CIt's%20deja%20vu%20all%20over,final%20game%20of%20the%20season.

Dawsey, J. (2018, January 12). Trump derides protections for immigrants from 'shithole' countries. *The Washington Post*. Retrieved February 25, 2018 from https://www.washingtonpost.com/politics/trump-attacks-protections-for-immigrants-from-shithole-countries-in-oval-office-meeting/2018/01/11/bfc0725c-f711-11e7-91af-31ac729add94_story.html?utm_term=.728b8708648a.

Faimberg, H. (2005). *The telescoping of generations: Listening to the narcissistic links between generations*. New York: Routledge.

Hollander, N. C. (2017). Who is the sufferer and what is being suffered? Subjectivity in times of social malaise. *Psychoanalytic Dialogues, 27*, 635–650.

Kennedy, M. (2018, March 9). ACLU sues ICE for allegedly separating 'hundreds' of migrant families. *National Public Radio*. Retrieved March 11, 2018 from https://www.npr.org/sections/thetwo-way/2018/03/09/592374637/aclu-sues-ice-for-allegedly-separating-hundreds-of-migrant-families.

Kifner, J. (1970, May 5). 4 Kent State students killed by troops. Retrieved January 20, 2025 from https://www.nytimes.com/1970/05/05/archives/4-kent-state-students-killed-by-troops-8-hurt-as-shooting-follows.html.

Lincoln, A. (1859, September 30). Address before the Wisconsin State Agricultural Society. Milwaukee, WI. Retrieved February 25, 2018 from http://www.abrahamlincolnonline.org/lincoln/speeches/fair.htm.

Nossiter, A., & Gladstone, R. (2015, November 13). Paris attacks kill more than 100, police say; Border controls tightened. Retrieved January 19, 2025 from https://www.nytimes.com/2015/11/14/world/europe/paris-shooting-attacks.html.

Samuels, A. (2017). The 'activist client': Social responsibility, the political self, and clinical practice in psychotherapy and psychoanalysis. *Psychoanalytic Dialogues, 27*, 678–693.

Spiegelman, A. (1986). *Maus: A survivor's tale: My father bleeds history*. New York: Pantheon Books.

Starr, K. E. (2008). *Repair of the soul: Metaphors of transformation in Jewish mysticism and psychoanalysis*. New York: Routledge.

Starr, K. E. (2018). Caught in the crossfire: Political intersections, collisions, and confrontations. *Psychoanalysis, Self, and Context, 13*, 389–397.

Thrush, G. (2017, March 6). Trump's new travel ban blocks migrants from six nations, sparing Iraq. *The New York Times*. Retrieved from https://www.nytimes.com/2017/03/06/us/politics/travel-ban-muslim-trump.html.

Uris, L. (1958). *Exodus*. New York: Doubleday.

Wang, A. B. (2018, January 24). Border patrol agents were filmed dumping water left for migrants: Then came a 'suspicious' arrest. *The Washington Post*. Retrieved March 11, 2018 from https://www.washingtonpost.com/news/post-nation/wp/2018/01/23/border-patrol-accused-of-targeting-aid-group-that-filmed-agents-dumping-water-left-for-migrants/?utm_term=.54dcd1c285b1.

Section 4

Hidden, Discovered, Evolved

Chapters by S. Pasternak, J. Kite, and M. Baker

Self-disclosure remains a controversial issue in psychoanalysis. Consequently, important personal experiences that have the potential to definitively shape new theoretical developments are typically sidelined or excluded from discussion. The development of theory or praxis is rarely connected to the personal history of our analytic mentors; nor have we many "first person" accounts that directly attribute the personal to theoretical advancements, or psychoanalytic technique. Biographical *backstories,* emerging from scholarly discovery, hypothesis, and conjecture raise the possibility of connection. For example, could Winnicott's idea of the "good enough" mother have something to do with his own childhood experience? Did the "dead mother complex" emerge from Andre Green's observations and the challenge of his own relationship? Is the well-known tortured connection between Melanie Klein and her mother the origin of her essential representation of the "good" and "bad" breast and her seminal exploration regarding the difficult integration of love and hate?

Psychobiography is the study of these connections. In 1977, *Faces in a Cloud* (Stolorow & Atwood, 1977) proposed that there are meaningful psychological origins to the metapsychology of Freud, Jung, Reik and Rank. Stolorow and Atwood argued that Freud's theory of psychosexual development may be "partially viewed as serving a defensive-restitutive effort by Freud to protect an idealized image of his mother against profound unconscious ambivalence" (Stolorow & Atwood, 1977, p. 48); that Jung's collective unconscious and archetypes are derived from early "secret childhood preoccupations" and "the danger of self-obliteration through absorption in fantasies of being devoured by omnipotent objects" (Stolorow & Atwood, 1977, p. 94). Stolorow and Atwood emphasized that the most significant understanding of theory occurs when it is "stripped of reifications and translated into its phenomenological terms" (Stolorow & Atwood, 1977, p. 107), an idea that we have applied to the understanding of everything, from presidents, dictators, scientists and artists, to ourselves.

In the world of psychoanalysis, there are some in our field whose openness has allowed us to see the threads of connection between a personal event, theoretical interest, and clinical praxis. Given his appreciation of

DOI: 10.4324/9781003584803-14

psychohistory, perhaps it is no surprise that Stolorow (2022) directly locates the idea of a "relational home" or "dwelling place for grief", (Stolorow, 2022, p. 139) to the traumatic loss of his daughter. Sensitive to the existential and its intersection with psychoanalysis and philosophy, Stolorow was already thinking about mortality and mourning, when other personal events pulled him further into his interrogation of finitude, trauma and loss.

Anna Ornstein's ideas about mourning, healing, and resilience have often been tied to her experience in Auschwitz and her survival of the Holocaust. In her personal memoir, *My Mother's Eyes* (Ornstein, 2004) – she speaks of her experience in vivid detail. And though perhaps a bit less personal than Stolorow in her analytic writing, Ornstein freely acknowledges the profound asset that a secure family life prior to loss, and access to a supportive community after loss, affects the resilience of trauma survivors and the capacity for mourning. There is no question where her perspective comes from, and this brings an additional integrity to her understanding of injury and healing.

In this final section, our contributors take what is unequivocally personal and reveal how it has shaped their ideas, their emotional comprehension of themselves, their praxis, and the creative consequences of their experience. They elevate our concepts of attunement and empathy and deepen our understanding of the events that shape who they are, and how we practice as psychoanalysts and psychotherapists. As they share their stories, we may consider how each has become a version of a psycho*auto*biographer – a person who has contributed in some way to the development of a theory, or praxis, by sharing a very personal experience, and reflecting on the way it has shaped how they think and their identity as clinicians. This is an opportunity to understand how their perspective, often derived from a definitive historical event, or meaningful personal focus, is considered over time, evolves, and becomes integrated into their identities.

Susan Pasternak shares her clinical experience with a challenging patient, whose intrusions into her personal life might have been the end of treatment, but instead evolved into a profound understanding of fragility, and an unusual and moving resolution – a ritual of mourning that reveals enormous power and personal authority. Jane V. Kite describes how her focus on the moral core of the analyst, and the concept of ethics in psychoanalysis grew out of a personal event that was impossible to ignore or to hide from the larger community. In a searing unfolding, she shares the challenge that she faced when her personal and professional life was abruptly and traumatically disrupted, and how the traumatic event shaped her formulation of the analyst's ethical unconscious. Michele Baker describes the intrusion of a personal medical decision that affected her clinical practice, and the different positions around self-disclosure with her patients. With the passage of time, and with the advantage of several ongoing dyads, she offers a unique opportunity to engage with her clients and reflect together on that time, how they understood their reactions to her news, and to their experience of the treatment, so many years ago, and now.

In each chapter, we are given the unique opportunity to encounter a vivid and personal reckoning in the clinical encounter, each highlighting the vivid differences and outcomes in the uniqueness of the therapeutic dyad, and the endlessly varied experience of self-disclosure by the clinician, and how these experiences shape each clinician's identity.

References

Ornstein, A. (2004). *My mother's eyes*. Clerisy Press, Emmis Books.
Stolorow, R., & Atwood, G. (1977). *Faces in a cloud subjectivity in personality theory*, Jason Aronson, Inc.
Stolorow, R. D. (2022). Faces of finitude: Death, loss, and trauma. *Psychoanalytic Inquiry, 42*, 135–140.

10 Dogmas, Difficulties, and Dilemmas

The Role of Self-Disclosure

Susan Pasternak

Most psychodynamic clinicians believe one of the most important ingredients of psychotherapy is to understand the uniqueness of the individual patient, and the uniqueness of the relationship that develops between patient and clinician. We are adept at describing theories of the mind and of technique, of the unconscious and its function, of transference phenomena and the role of the past and the presence of conflict; but we have been less successful in our explanations of our encounters with analytic dogma, and the difficulties and dilemmas that arise, with even the most experienced clinician.

For 30 years I taught a weekly seminar, *Dogmas, Dilemmas, and Difficulties or Questions to Which We Should Know the Answers* to psychiatrists, psychoanalytic candidates, and psychologists. Over the years, our discussions were poignant, funny, insightful, and intelligent, and included profoundly thoughtful questions. I continue to be grateful to those who came and shared their frank concerns. I am certain it improved my work and my teaching as well.

At the beginning of the seminar, I would ask the attendees to list questions that they would like to address. We then shuffled these questions into categories, and, interestingly, these categories inevitably were the same every year: Taboos, physical contact, self-disclosure, gratification, gifts, mistakes, money, parameters of the hour, sexual feelings for both doctor and patients, physical illness of both patient and doctor, death and suicide. I am going to focus on self-disclosure which I believe can overlap with the category of gratification.

At the beginning of each seminar, I assigned a well-known article by Jody Davies (1994) in which a male patient in the course of the treatment asked if she, Dr. Davies, were flirting with him. Dr. Davies stated, "I believe I am". Dr. Davies' response acknowledged her own awareness of, and reaction to, her patient's sexuality – a self-disclosing response. In that specific treatment Dr. Davies argued that the validation of adult sexuality is not sufficiently explored either in the analytic literature or in treatment. In other words, clinicians tend to look at their patient's sexuality as pre-oedipal/childhood issues and that erotic transference, while challenging to many clinicians, also represents an aspect of healthy adult desire that is important to explore. Dr. Davies believed that what she said to the patient had helped him recognize and own his adult sexuality and uncover his paralyzing inhibitions. But it's not easy to go there!

DOI: 10.4324/9781003584803-15

Some attendees wondered if it would not have been better to have transferred the patient to another clinician due to the sexual implication. Others believed that, ultimately, it was useful, but noted that they could not imagine responding that way. Additional responses included questions such as: Was it transference/counter transference? Was it a boundary violation to tell your patient about your attraction? Is it bad? Is it ok? I believe that answers to these kinds of questions must ideally be on the side of what is helpful to the patient – as long as it remains within ethical boundaries. Can the patient and analyst tolerate exploring these feelings that may be accessed *in that moment*? How might we understand those feelings and translate them into meaningful content and relevant communication, while maintaining the connection and alliance. Our determination of the best outcome for the patient is not always clear. If we self-disclose (i.e., gratify), do we foreclose a deeper understanding that particular patient's needs because we have collapsed the limits? Or we also might hypothesize the exact opposite if we do not answer. In either case, how do we make the therapy effective?

When a patient asks personal questions, it is easier for some clinicians to turn the question around and ask why it is important to know, or what it would mean to know – in other words to fall back on the rule of abstinence. All these dogmas, dilemmas, and difficulties so easily can become polarized between the perception of the right way or the wrong way to treat a patient– I believe that each clinician must try to understand their feelings about self-disclosure in that moment and with that patient. What is my patient trying to express to me and me to the patient and how together do we understand this?

If I am not comfortable answering a question I will say so, indicating that the problem is mine, not theirs for asking. The responses to this are varied: anger, disappointment, or even, understanding. If I hear that maybe the question could be about something else, I will inquire. Yet I have come to see that it is more common for me to answer personal questions than not, questions that seek out my thoughts and feelings relevant to what is going on at that time in the treatment. As such, I must reflect that I am responding because it is difficult not to, that I have concerns about the patient's hurt or anger, or evidence of dislike, or rejection of the treatment itself. In these moments, the question of self-disclosure becomes a meaningful way to use oneself – ones revealing thoughts, impressions and feeling – in the service of the treatment, to understand the many needs that are in play. The self-disclosure dilemma can be understood as overlapping with the concept of gratification of the patient, and the analyst.

Clinical Example

In the late 1980s, the issue of self-disclosure was laid bare by one of the most difficult challenges of my career. Facts regarding the patient have been altered to protect his identity. Mr. P. had been referred to me following numerous attempts to locate "the right" therapist. Mr. P., a 26-year-old gay man, had recently moved with his partner from the West Coast. He was unemployed and living off the substantial salary of his partner, an arrangement that caused friction between the two men.

When I first saw him sitting outside my office, I observed an attractive man, with a chiseled jaw line, that I was later told had been cosmetically reconstructed. He had bleached hair and wore a cape over a tee shirt and tight blue jeans. His superhero attire evoked Batman or Superman.

I had the impulse to giggle but contained myself. Who was this caped young man? He swept into my office and immediately proceeded to tell me that he did not want to work but aimed to attend school, though he was unsure of his focus. Mr. P. was clearly intelligent; he had aspired to be a doctor, but believed he would flunk premed classes because he was so undisciplined. He also told me that he was HIV positive and was being treated in Paris by one of the original HIV researchers. I wondered about the veracity of this story, though it turned out to be true. Mr. P. had been prescribed a large cocktail of experimental medications, and his T-cell count remained high. But Mr. P. was very concerned about his health – acknowledging that survival from AIDS was rare. In our first hour, he told me that if he became very sick, he refused to die an ugly, humiliating death and would suicide with an overdose of barbiturates.

When Mr. P. left my office, I was aware of his need for control and apparent sense of entitlement; beneath his flamboyance, and understandable concern about his health was a palpable vulnerability. His adamant stance about killing himself if he got very sick was terrifying to me because, on one hand, I felt I must do everything I could to prevent it and on the other, I understood that he did not want to die the agonizing death from AIDS of so many young men. Though death permeated his world, Mr. P. adamantly resisted talking about his own mortality throughout the years of our work together. When I tried to ask him if he could tell me why he didn't want to talk about this, he refused.

Something about this patient tapped into my own narcissism. To be chosen by him after so much therapist shopping, I felt compelled to be careful, not to disappoint. What does it mean to be anointed by a clever shopper and what effect does that have on the therapy? I think it is important that we ask ourselves these kinds of questions. Mr. P. wanted a therapist who could understand things on "a deep level", but what he really seemed to want was supportive therapy with only a tincture of psychodynamic work.

I quickly learned about his childhood. Mr. P. had come from an affluent family. During his first 11 years, his father, while climbing the corporate ladder of a large company, moved the family at least seven times. Mr. P.'s mother was a housewife. He had three sisters. We talked a great deal about the many moves and how he felt like an outsider and different. Later those feelings turned into a belief that something was wrong with him.

Those early years seemed to blur into one painful memory of humiliation. He thought that the bad feelings began in 1st grade with one painful event. During the day at school he had spent a great deal of time cutting out and coloring a bright smiling yellow sun that he put around his neck. Even his teacher admired his beautiful creation. It was as if he had his own personal sun warming him and smiling at him. He felt less alone. He wore the sun necklace onto the school bus – proud of his artwork. When he was about to board, the bus monitor took the sun and crushed it in her hands, then said, "Get that stupid grin off your face". He never understood the action of this woman, nor did I, but he felt humiliated and crushed just like that sun. Mr. P. believed that that event was a metaphor for a large part of his life – that anything that he did or felt good about would be ruined, so why bother. He was quite convincing, and my eyes filled with tears. I acknowledged how painful it must have been. In my own training there was a dogma: a therapist never cries in front of a patient. As I sat with him, feeling sad and aghast at my own wet eyes, I realized I had broken a "rule". Then Mr. P. began to sob. He cried then for the first and only time in the nearly ten years I saw him. He cried unashamedly for that very sad 1st grade little boy. He remembered that moment with me and referred to it as a time he felt understood as never before.

Mr. P.'s parents had been distant. He conveyed the sense that he was physically well taken care of, but not emotionally. When he came out to them, they were very disapproving; over time they accepted their son's homosexuality but not his flamboyant lifestyle. Mr. P. was not especially close to his two older sisters, converts to a rigid form of Christianity. Their intolerance infuriated him and he would unleash his wrath upon them with biting criticism, a defensive style that diminished only somewhat as the treatment progressed. His awareness of my more open response to him was in striking difference to his experience with his parents and siblings. While I do not advocate crying with a patient, I believe that the dogma that therapists should avoid, or never show emotion, needs to be examined through the lens of each unique relationship, and that the withholding of affect by the analyst can sometimes resonate with unnecessary pain. Often, I felt like a mother listening to a little boy reporting the day's events. But I did not interpret the maternal transference. I believed that to acknowledge and validate what he was feeling and telling me would do more to further and deepen our work than if I clarified or interpreted. On the infrequent occasion when I would trot out some interpretation, he would listen, nod, maybe yawn, or shake his head and continue what he was saying. Once in a while, Mr. P. would surprise me by affirming an analytic comment.

Throughout our work together, Mr. P. and his partner traveled to exotic places on fabulous trips. His impressions and observations of his journeys interested me deeply, and over time, his behavior on the trips seemed to reflect his growth and deepening introspection. At first, he would regale me with stories of outlandish behavior – how he would describe himself to whomever he met that he was a Swiss count or a well-published physician. His stories could be extremely funny. Later in our work he became aware that his trips were a moment in time when he could pretend that he was important and famous. I believe that my genuine interest in and curiosity about his travels, helped fuel his motivation to explore what his behavior meant.

Eventually, Mr. P′ decided he would go to nursing school, since medical school was not realistic. Doing well physically, he was greatly validated by his academic choice, although there were still difficult moments of dangerous acting out including two brief psychiatric hospitalizations. He continued to allow himself to see that his grandiosity came from feelings of self-hatred, and he became much more tolerant when I held up the psychological mirror to him. A little to my unspoken disappointment, he gave up his costume of capes. Mr. P. graduated first in his nursing school class – a proud moment for everyone – and took a good job in a hospital. Things seemed to go more smoothly.

We had been working together for nearly seven years. At this point, Mr. P. began to bring gifts from his travels. One of the difficulties that comes up in the dogmas, difficulties and dilemmas context is how respond to these offerings. Can we receive gifts – can we give gifts? Though the taboo of accepting an extravagant gift is clearly not ethical, issues around smaller ones seem less so. After one of his vacations, Mr. P. brought me chocolate bars. Had an inadvertent self–disclosure tipped him off? I am ashamed to say, he probably caught me hastily chewing a chocolate as we began a session. He also gave me a very small, inexpensive replica of a Hindu carving, as well as some small travel brochures from his trips to India. I would express my appreciation of his thoughtfulness and might inquire how he had decided to bring me those specific objects. We spent a great deal of time talking about what India meant to him and his wish to have his ashes scattered over the Ganges when he died.

Toward the end of his first year working as a nurse, I was diagnosed with breast cancer. Again, that dilemma of self-disclosure: How much do we, should we, can we disclose to our patients? Do we tell our patients about our illnesses, particularly when the illness will lead to a relatively long absence? Is it a burden for them? Is it important for certain patients to know? Is it too painful for others to know and what are the reasons for each?

At the time of my diagnosis, I was uncertain what to share with my patients. I tried to think about what was best for me and for them; I sought consultation and decided, in the end, that my desire for privacy outweighed anything else. In other words, it was okay to do what I wanted for myself. I told all my patients only that I was taking a medical leave for six weeks to have surgery. What I did do was explore the meaning of the absence and asked them what they imagined was wrong. There was a great deal of useful therapeutic interaction. Interestingly, I was relieved and even surprised to realize that the non-disclosure of any other details appeared acceptable to all of us. No one asked about a diagnosis. It strongly suggested to me, in retrospect, that I had inadvertently vaccinated them against asking specific questions about the reason for my absence, what might be going on, and what it might mean.

As I look back, I believe in some unconscious way my patients were responding to and respecting my wish not to tell them any details; though I asked about their feelings and fantasies, and even if they feared I might die, I believe my response to the situation was counterphobic. I also believe that most, but not all, felt my genuine concern about their well-being for the six weeks I would be away.

Many colleagues and students have asked if I would do it differently now, should the situation present itself to me again. On reflection, I might. I might tell my patients what was wrong depending on each individual patient. Perhaps I can say this now, after a full recovery; but I believe that at the time, my own narcissistic vulnerabilities were packed into the mix. Some I was aware of and others I did not want to look at.

When I told Mr. P. about my surgery and the absence, he was seemingly uncurious, his usual way of behaving. You can imagine my surprise when many months after the surgery, he came into the session and told me that he had a confession to make. Mr. P. said, "Every day after you left for surgery, I went up to the OR to see what surgery was scheduled for the day. I found yours and so I have known for a long time that you had breast cancer". He told me that he knew my husband worked at the same hospital as he. He knew we lived in Cambridge and had two young children. At that time there were no HIPAA rules to be violated, but my privacy had been breached. So much for my non-disclosure.

I have presented this case many times over many years. The most common response from colleagues was that they found this patient's behavior a very aggressive, egregious, and disrespectful intrusion and would transfer the patient to someone else. Others stated that, though the behavior was extremely inappropriate, they would try to work with the patient to understand the motivation for this behavior. Some found my response therapeutic. Of course, my blind spots could have interfered with these reactions, but in truth, his confession moved me. Yes, it would have been more direct had he told me much earlier. He said that he knew it was a "shameful" thing to do, but now he felt so much closer to me. I was more similar to him: I knew what it was to face the possibility of death. The revelation occurred at the same time as his T cell count was dropping and he was contending with a persistent dry cough. I am sure this fueled the intensity of his behavior.

I surprised myself that I was so moved that this "boy man" went to such desperate lengths to know what was wrong with me. It was not his behavior, but my feelings in reaction to his behavior, that guided me. I used the feelings to locate my perspective, his perspective, and then together we looked at the underpinnings of what had motivated him.

He believed that my experience would allow me to more deeply understand the lethality of his illness, and expressed happiness that I was alive, and was there to be with him during his own trials. I continued to work with him, to sort through the practicalities of his illness while continuing to respect his powerful refusal to not engage in issues of his unavoidable mortality.

We continued our work for two and a half more years, during which time Mr. P. became more and more symptomatic, but still managed to come to therapy. The last time I saw Mr. P., he was very ill with an opportunistic pneumonia and was desperately trying to find a new study and access to another

AIDS drug. After the session we said we would see each other the following week. The morning before our next scheduled appointment, I received a call from his father telling me that Mr. P. had taken a very large overdose of barbiturates and "was finally at peace surrounded by his Hindu artifacts".

His father asked if I would come to the memorial service. Such a request raises many of the dogmas, dilemmas, and difficulties that have been discussed. To make matters even more complex, there is a postscript. As mentioned earlier, Mr. P. wanted to have his ashes scattered over the Ganges. He committed suicide in the end of November. Absolutely coincidentally, I was going to India with my family for a long-planned vacation. I still believe there was no possible way that the patient could have known about that trip. I decided to tell Dr. P.'s father of my upcoming plans, and I offered to bring his son's ashes to India to fulfill Dr. P.'s long-standing wish. At the funeral Mr. P.'s parents presented me with a beautiful glass bottle holding a portion of his ashes. Several weeks later in the city of Varanasi, as the sun was rising, I scattered Mr. P.'s ashes on the Ganges.

When, over the years, I have shared this decision with colleagues, I have been met with a myriad of responses: that my offer was a serious boundary crossing, and an over involvement with the patient. There have been expressions of disbelief and astonishment, as well as understanding. In this case I strongly believed that no boundaries were crossed, because the patient was not alive. Was I over involved? Was it inappropriate? All the questions and concerns that were raised have allowed me to reflect and examine myself.

There are still so many ways to try to think about what happened. Must we do absolutely everything we can to keep our suicidal patients alive, and could I have prevented his action? If I could have, would I have? Did my patient feel that I had I given up on him or did his imminent mortality, change my responsibility? What about taking the ashes to India? Was I taking them for atonement, for forgiveness? Out of guilt, out of respect?

My technique regarding self-disclosure has evolved since I began treating patients 40 years ago. Have the various psychodynamic teaching institutions also evolved? I have come to believe that there is no codified cookbook answers to the enormously varied and complex dynamics that arise in psychotherapy and psychoanalysis, and I hope that most institutions share that belief. We can be guided by closely attending to our patients' uniqueness and the important emotional subtext that we bring as clinicians. We can be aided in this task by actively confronting the dogmas, dilemmas, and difficulties that inevitably arise in work that is unique and, like life itself, is inherently uncertain.

Reference

Davies, J. M. (1994). Love in the afternoon: A relational reconsideration of desire and dread in the countertransference. *Psychoanalytic Dialogues*, *4*(2), 153–170.

11 What Can't I Say? Sexual Boundary Violations and Ethics in Psychoanalysis

Jane V. Kite

Following an in-person presentation in 2023 on the subject of the analyst's self-disclosure, I write here about two related threads in our field that get very little concerted attention because they fall largely outside the realm of established theory in psychoanalysis: sexual trauma and ethics. Although these threads are intimately related, I think you'll agree that they appear most often as loose ends, two realms that we approach in concert only when we have to. I'll be approaching these related threads via my personal experience of the trauma associated with a sexual boundary violation, and trace where that ultimately took me theoretically. I'll also attempt briefly to link this experience to the conceptual confusions we encounter in thinking about and attempting to teach ethics in psychoanalysis.

I was pleased to have been asked to present at the APsA discussion group ("Facing the Facts: Self-Disclosure and the Analytic Relationship"), but I can say now that I was also anxious about it. The heart of the self-disclosure in my case – the account of a sexual boundary violation that upended my life – is something we don't talk about much if at all in our field, given the fact that the history of psychoanalysis is rife with it, or perhaps *because* the history of our field is rife with it. Some facts are uniquely hard to face.

A more forthright way to say this might be that the beginning of my interest in ethics in psychoanalysis was frankly traumatic. In 2009, I found out – stumbled upon, really – the fact that my husband, a well-known analyst, had been having an in-office sexual relationship with a patient for well over a year. Our offices were in our home. Needless to say, I was devastated, and speechless. In fact, I wasn't "allowed" to speak about it with anyone for several months, as strenuous attempts were made to cover it up. I was quite literally silenced. In fact, the situation didn't become public knowledge for almost a year, when a court reporter with access to testimony after the patient sued, published a detail-laden story in an underground newspaper that rapidly spread through the local community. The testimony-based details of what had happened were salacious; horrifying, actually. I was mentioned by name in the article, on the basis of which my name became permanently linked to his on the internet. It still is, if you go back far enough.

DOI: 10.4324/9781003584803-16

The salacious story was quickly taken down, but the damage was done. Even though – or perhaps because this was all supposed to be confined to "rumor and innuendo", as we typically say in our flight from what happened, our irreparably fractured local community still couldn't talk about it, and legal constraints prevented me from talking about it with anyone. Nor did I really want to; I was ashamed. Patients continued with him in analysis, many of them ignorant of what had happened. Some were intentionally misinformed, told "it was a supervisee, not a patient", for instance. The idea of truth was almost laughably absent at that point. What did it mean for me to be an analyst in this mess? Could I continue as if "nothing" had happened?

Now I'm thinking, almost 15 years later, "should I even be telling you this much?" Am I burdening you? Should there be limits to self-revelation? I realize that I'm directly communicating the "too muchness" characteristic of trauma here, particularly sexual trauma. Ellen Pinsky has observed (private communication) that the boundary violations literature emphasizes the dilemma of the analyst while neglecting the harm to the patient and the profession. Much of what had happened was literally unspeakable in the professional community in Boston, and much of what I felt personally was doubly unspeakable, frankly guilt-producing. The worst thing that had ever befallen me (and there were significant early traumas in my "worst things" category) was off limits; I was forbidden to talk about the details with anyone. My trauma became an encysted affect, a feeling that was with me constantly, but had to remain mute.

The personal repercussions of this episode continued. The fact that my name was now permanently linked to that of my soon to be ex-husband on the internet proved to be disastrous. Patients of mine who found out about it left my practice, firmly convinced that I must have known about this all along, and was part of a conspiracy to cover it up. My husband and I had been practicing in the same house after all – how could I not have known? Referrals stopped. One patient of mine who had been sexually abused as a child by a family member found the online account and became actively psychotic, threatening to sue me, and left treatment abruptly after ten years of committed and painstaking analysis. This was heartbreaking. The impact of my husband's transgression was far-reaching. What could I say, and how could others approach me? My personal life had shattered, and the foundations of my professional life were badly shaken. There was no recourse. I did go back into analysis, which helped re-establish a floor under me. My analyst was the only person I could speak openly with.

Ultimately, when I could think again, I began to think and to write about ethics. The short version of what I have to say today is that I began thinking seriously about ethics in psychoanalysis because I had to; what felt like a nuclear bomb had gone off in my life, and I had to find a way to think about it that went beyond myself. My conviction as an analyst has always been that the engine of our work starts in autobiography, to which I would now add the singular significance of nodal traumas. The personal. The sexual boundary violation in my life had hit me and my institute like a meteorite, leaving what felt like a smoking crater and a group of zombies in its wake. It had been literally *unthinkable* at the time. I was among those whose *inner* lives had been indelibly altered, yet who seemed to have no *direct* claim to harm.

Gradually, I began thinking about psychoanalytic theory, and what it does and doesn't address in terms of trauma, and what we might call moral injury. I came to the uneasy conclusion that the maelstrom that follows a traumatic sexual transgression is linked to an enduring fault line in our field, and that is our relative silence around trauma in general and sexual trauma in particular.

A couple of years ago at a virtual national meeting, a colleague who was apparently alluding to our psychoanalytic ancestry, spontaneously slipped and said, "incestry". It was barely noticed. I noticed it, because it captured precisely what I might call our ethical trouble as a field, starting with Freud's *unavowal*, in Erik Erikson's terms (1976), of sexual trauma in the form of incest, and the subsequent bifurcation of trauma theories on the one hand, and theories of unconscious conflict on the other.

Material reality and psychical reality had been initially parsed out in psychoanalysis with what appeared to be Freud's radical retreat from his early seduction theory in 1897. It was here that traumatic experience – specifically sexual trauma and incest – was sidelined as the probable cause of neurotic illness in favor of the workings of unconscious fantasy. His rationale, now famous, but still ill-understood, was "the fact that in every case the father, not excluding my own, had to be blamed as a pervert" (Freud, 1896, p. 259). This in turn is linked to "the certain insight that because there are no indications of reality in the unconscious, it is impossible to distinguish between truth and fiction cathected with affect" (Freud, 1896, p. 260).

"Fiction cathected with affect" (fantasy, allegedly) proved to be a preternaturally sturdy characterization of distress in women. While manifestly true in some cases, "fiction cathected with affect" was a fatefully ambiguous distinction, and one with echoes that persist to this day. I'll break in here to say that this formulation is the common ancestor of the #MeToo movement, and uncomfortably close to our tendency to dismiss allegations of sexual trauma in particular as "fiction cathected with affect", or, in institute life, the requisite "rumor and innuendo". We can't know what "really" happened. Similarly, I believe that in reflexively turning away from the trauma of sexual boundary violations – incest in our field – we repeat Freud's pivot from his early seduction hypothesis to a theory of fantasy and unconscious conflict as the nidus of neurotic illness. With this move, traumatic sexual experience is sidelined, potentially alchemized as hearsay, as fantasy; one quick step from incest to Oedipus. Ethics, on the other hand, relies on clarifying the *difference* between reality and fantasy.

In fact, as I began to explore it, I found that the concept of ethics, while commonly assumed as central in our praxis, is not a psychoanalytic concept and remains riddled with conceptual confusion in our field. The one entry under "Ethics" in the index to the Standard Edition says "see Morality", with which it is routinely conflated. A few months before his now famous letter to Fliess in September of 1897, Freud had written in a memorandum that "incest is anti-social and civilization consists in a radical renunciation of it" (Freud, 1897, memorandum to Fleiss). By history and currently, I argue that incest in the form of sex with patients is the index trauma in our field; anti-social, uncivilized, an unbearable excess. Incest is also an unburied ancestor in psychoanalysis; it haunts our field. Never laid to rest, incest is spun into theory obliquely via the myth of Oedipus, where it has an eerie half-life in the form of unwitting sex with a parent. But at the same time, incest in the form of sex between analyst and patient in the practice of psychoanalysis *isn't* a myth, and it isn't "unwitting", it is real – an eruption of *the* Real in Lacan's terms, an unbearable excess, the "primal crime" according to Muriel Dimen (2016). Typically voluble, we analysts become speechless in the face of incest in our field. Failures of this kind in analysis aren't experienced, but dissociated.

Peter Rudnytsky, quoting Bohleber in his recent book *Mutual Analysis* (Rudnytsky, 2022), an in-depth exploration of Ferenczi's work and the origins of trauma theory, writes: "In the same way that traumatic *experience* forms a kind of dissociated foreign body in the psychic-associative network of an individual, so too trauma theory has functioned as a "dissociated foreign body" in the psychic-associative network of psychoanalysis" (Rudnytsky, 2022, p. 20). I agree with him. He also mentions Bennett Simon (1992), whose ingenious paper ironically entitled "Incest, see under Oedipus Complex", captures what he calls our "split brain" approach to incest. "In a way that is analogous to the defenses used by survivors of incest", Simon writes, "psychoanalysis has both known and not known, avowed and disavowed, the traumatic impact of actual abuse" (Simon, 1992, p. 962).

I began to think that with each incestuous crisis in our institutes, we inadvertently reenact Freud's early *unavowal* of his seduction theory and actual incest, and move toward what Joyce Slochower has aptly called "the loneliness of trauma's absent historicity and accountability" (Slochower, 2021, p. 152). Those of us who know what happened struggle to speak. I couldn't speak. That I'm speaking to you now still feels forbidden. Patients in our offices struggle to speak about incest in their own backgrounds, an experience which has often been dissociated, and remains wordless. Incest in our field remains largely wordless.

Furthermore, in a way that's directly analogous to the aftermath of parent/child incest, the institute and indeed the *profession itself* becomes the confused child in relation to the "sexuality of the mad adult" in Ferenczi's terms in his classic paper "Confusion of Tongues between Adults and the Child" (1933a) in the wake of sexual misconduct in one of its members (pp. 156–67). Candidates, who are still speaking the language of tenderness early in training, are violently let down. We all scatter. It is impossible for any of us to think freely, let alone speak freely, about what has happened. In fact, sexual trauma and incest in institutes is *routinely* dissociated; it is literally unthinkable. At the same time, it directly signifies the abiding ethical fragility woven into the fabric of our profession. With sexual trauma at our institutes, we are suddenly snapped back in time to some of the earliest debates in our field over the impact of actual sexual trauma and incest, and the reflexive desire to cover it up and move on. Ancestry becomes *incestry* at these junctures. The ghosts of our histories, personal and professional, resurface to haunt us. We have to suffer rather than live our ethics.

It is clear that sexually transgressive analysts aren't aware of the unconscious, typically traumatic determinants involved in misusing a patient. They don't know in any direct way what a transgressive parent, a neglectful parent, a depriving parent, a sexually seductive parent may have contributed to their own actions. Furthermore, like a bewildered Oedipus entangled in his own destiny, they don't *know* that they don't know what they're doing. They don't know that what they are visiting upon their patient is usually a fantastically complex, disguised version of what was visited upon them until it is too late. I'll add parenthetically here that it is Laplanche who highlights the fact that it is the rigidities and inadequacies in our theories which "allow sexual crime to slip away" (Laplanche, 2011, p. 155).

Sexual crime in psychoanalysis slips away because it is unspeakable and untheorizable. "Sexual boundary violations" have everything to do with the analyst's unconscious functioning, their own infantile sexuality, and nothing to do with didactic instruction. For me, as I've written elsewhere, the inescapable conclusion is that the ethical both resides and gets lost with the person of the analyst in what I am calling the gap: the characteristic, largely *unconscious* way in which the individual analyst practices (Kite, 2016). Ethics as an abstraction is useless. It has to have everything to do with real life, and how we live it.

So how do we "teach" ethics in psychoanalytic institutes? I would argue that we can't, actually, because the ethical is always *lived*, and lived in a way that is out of awareness. Even though we may have wished for a focus on ethics from the beginning of training, ethics in psychoanalysis has everything to do with the analyst's unconscious functioning, and very little to do with didactic instruction. Fundamentally, that is, our ethics are unconscious, yet alive in everything we do. Ethics can be described as the mute unconscious roadmaps of our earliest object relations, mapping how we've been treated, loved or unloved, by others, and how we reflexively position ourselves in relation to others. Our ethics as individuals remain largely unconscious, yet hopefully revealed, at least partially, in our own analyses via what we come to know about ourselves. Typically, we don't really think much about the foundational role ethics plays in our work with others – our actions as analysts – until we have to; until, that is, something unequivocally *un*ethical has happened. A more immediate apprehension of ethics in analytic practice doesn't begin with ethics courses, but with the radical eruption of forgotten, suppressed, or disavowed traumatic experiences in the analyst. Sexual boundary violations are Exhibit A in this arena. These eruptions are abrupt reminders that psychoanalysis as a formal discipline is most consequentially based in what is *not* known in either member of the couple, and that this "not known" in the analyst in particular has profound ethical implications. The idea of ethics as we begin to scrutinize it undoes all of our neat conceptual categories, and routinely destabilizes any certainty we may have about the fundamental integrity of psychoanalytic work.

I have argued in an earlier paper (Kite, 2016) that it is *precisely* what remains unknown *in the analyst* that is both the ethical foundation for our field and the locus of our resistance to the idea. We don't do well as a group with not knowing, especially when it comes to ourselves. We tend to pose as fully self-aware. Absent the familiar hideouts of our conceptual language – resistance, transference, countertransference – we have trouble remaining aware of ourselves in an immediate way in the consulting room. Wasn't that task wrapped up by the end of our own analyses we ask? I argue that it's not that analysts have to consciously conform to a higher moral standard than anyone else, but that we, like others, are largely unaware of the ethical basis for our relatedness to begin with. Our ethics as individuals are unconscious, as unique as a fingerprint.

My early fascination with analysis was abruptly curtailed by my intimate experience of this boundary violation. Living through it, however, has radically increased my appreciation for the potential reach of psychoanalysis, and the challenges posed by its theory. It has also caused me to question "ethics" as a cornerstone in psychoanalysis. We take ethics for granted as the basis of our practice, as Scarfone (2017) has pointed out, but we actually practice basically as ourselves, relying largely on what I have called our mute internal roadmaps, the unconscious reach of what we can't remember or can't know. This is a challenging arrangement, and one that calls for continued attention in our field.

I remain grateful for the opportunity to speak openly about what I might characterize as "a horribly important time in my life".

Bibliography

Dimen, M. (2016). Rotten apples and ambivalence: Sexual boundary violations through a psychocultural lens. *Journal of the American Psychoanalytic Association, 64*, 361–373.

Erikson, E. H. (1976). Psychoanalysis and ethics – avowed and unavowed. *International Review of Psychoanalysis, 3*, 409–414.

Ferenczi, S. (1933a). Confusion of tongues between adults and the child: The language of tenderness and of passion. In M. Balint (Ed.), *Final contributions to the methods and problems of psychoanalysis*. Trans. Ernest Jones (pp. 156–167). London: Forgotten Books, 2012.

Freud, S. (1896). The aetiology of hysteria. In *The standard edition of the complete psychological works of Sigmund Freud* (Vol. 1, 1886–1899). Letter 69, p. 259.

Freud, S. (1897). Letter from Freud to Fliess, September 21, 1897. *The complete letters of Sigmund Freud to Wilhelm Fliess*, 1887–1904. 42, 264–267.

Kite, J. (2016). The fundamental ethical ambiguity of the analyst as person. *Journal of the American Psychoanalytic Association, 64*, 1153–1171.

Laplanche, J. (2011). *Freud and the sexual*. International Psychoanalytic Books.

Rudnytsky, P. L. (2022). *Mutual analysis: Ferenczi, Severn, and the origins of trauma theory*. Routledge.
Scarfone, D. (2017). That is not psychoanalysis: Ethics as the main tool for psychoanalytic knowledge and discussion. *Psychoanalytic Dialogues, 27*, 392–400.
Simon, B. (1992). 'Incest – see under oedipus complex': The history of an error in psychoanalysis. *Journal of the American Psychoanalytic Association, 40*, 955–988.
Slochower, J. (2021). Don't tell anyone. In C. Levin (Ed.), *Sexual boundary trouble in psychoanalysis* (p. 152). Routledge.

12 Labyrinth[1]

Michele Baker

In 2014, I first presented the material I will revisit in this paper. Five years had passed since the surgery that is the subject of my disclosure. Now, it's been 15 years. As I reread my initial writeup, not only did I get to see my younger self's point of view, but I also had the chance to revisit my exchanges with the four patients I had written about. Because I still work with all four patients, I decided to include them in the second round of writing by asking them to share what my disclosure had meant to them. I asked each of them permission to share both the story of my initial disclosure and also details of our request discussions. All of them affirmatively agreed to do so, generously sharing their experiences. In 2014, I described how I disclosed. Now, in 2025, I'll add to that discussion how my patients felt about the disclosure.

In the following pages, I report three vignettes relatively briefly and then discuss a fourth story at somewhat greater length. I conclude with some ideas I've contemplated since revisiting my self-disclosure. Even though I had thought about my choices about disclosure as purposefully as I could in the context of the surgery I had in 2009, discussions with patients had felt to some degree unexpected and even inexplicable. What surprised me when I discussed how disclosure had unfolded with each of these four patients was how well the choices we made fit within our co-created dynamics.

I had the first of several prophylactic and reconstructive surgeries in July 2009. I had known that I had the BRCA1 mutation common in Ashkenazi Jews since 1999, ten years before my initial surgery, and I had not been originally planning to have prophylactic mastectomies. I had chosen close surveillance for the decade during which I got married and had my two children. But then I learned something that scared me deeply. Even with the most aggressive protocol of ultrasounds and MRIs, 4% of cases of breast cancer in women with a gene mutation are already metastatic at the time of diagnosis. I was becoming increasingly afraid of leaving my kids motherless. I scheduled surgery for July 2009 to minimize the disruption to my kids' schooling and to my work schedule. I planned to be out for a month, from mid-July through mid-August. It seemed that most patients assumed I'd be on vacation when I told them about my summer schedule. I didn't correct them. The patients who may have had other ideas about why I'd be away for a month didn't say so,

DOI: 10.4324/9781003584803-17

and I didn't push them to share. Perhaps patients read my wish for privacy (a wish that was especially intense in the time just before the surgery when I was so filled with angst) and colluded with me by staying mum.

As I limped back to the office after my month away, barely able to achieve an upright position, I knew it would be difficult to hide the fact that something drastic had happened to me. I had gone through a time of significant pain and I was still hurting and exhausted. I had lost almost 20 pounds over the course of a few weeks. I tried to figure out ahead of time what I would say to patients, assuming they would all exclaim some variant of "what the hell happened to you?!" But my planning was not particularly helpful. Most people didn't ask anything except, "how was your vacation?" The patients who hinted or asked each did so in idiosyncratic ways. Going back through my analytic process notes and other chart notes from that time allowed me to see how distinct each series of communications had been.

Before I had this experience, I had imagined that decisions about disclosure would depend most upon the character of the therapist/analyst and the specifics of the issue being disclosed. To my surprise, I found that the intersubjective space influenced by the patient's dynamics and my own was more influential in determining what I disclosed. Instead of acting independently forearmed with a particular intention to disclose or not, I ended up feeling my way through with each patient as a partner. Each patient brought an entirely novel subjectivity to our interactions, and I had less control over my own mind than I had imagined I would.

Jess

There were two patients I talked to about my surgeries soon after returning from my leave: both had been long-term twice-weekly therapy patients. The first patient I told, at some point shortly after the surgery, was a woman my age, a lesbian, with Post-traumatic stress disorder (PTSD) and depression. I think I told her because I suspected that she wouldn't be disgusted by my mastectomy. She had long had some gender dysphoria and had the wish that she could, as she put it, "cut off" her breasts. It was a relief to tell someone whom I knew wouldn't pity me. Also, early in our work together I had asked her about her childhood sexual abuse, but she would not discuss it unless I told her whether I had been molested. I had declined to answer, and true to her initial word, she had never shared details.

In the spring of 2025, I asked Jess if she would be willing to participate in a conversation about my self-disclosure. In our conversation, she confirmed my long-held impressions.

Me: In retrospect, what was my self-disclosure like for you?

Jess: Well, I mean, you know that I've always struggled with this whole idea that things have to be so separated. I was trying to deal with a few different things–I had to deal with the fact that I was suicidal. I don't really open up to most people at all. For me, it's always been a question of trust. It's one of those "I'll show you mine if you show me yours" kind of things.

Me: Would it be fair to say then, that me telling you this personal information was helpful to you?

Jess: Well, yeah, and it's also helpful because it would definitely change our dynamic if you didn't look the same and didn't acknowledge why, especially if you happened to know that I would gladly chop mine off, and, you know, put a tattoo over the top–I wouldn't even bother with the nipples. Screw the nipples, you know?

Me: So, it's not only "I'll show you mine if you show me yours", but it's also that you're not going to do well if your reality is denied?

Jess: I see with my own eyes, and if you're blank about that, that's going to be another blocker to me being able to feel comfortable. Yeah, 'cause I mean, one of my issues has always been that I couldn't tell anyone what happened to me when I was a kid.

Me: Yeah.

Jess: You're not just my doctor. You're not my PCP, you know? I'm supposed to talk to you not just about the things that are going on in my body, but actually what's going on in my mind.

Me: Was there any downside for you?

Jess: I think I was jealous. My boobs get in the way. They have always been in the way.

I did a whole bunch of jumps when I was skateboarding and especially when I was rollerblading and the thing is that sometimes you land on your front. And also, not to have to deal with your uterus–they tidy everything up down there. I was just like: I want that. I'm probably more of a guy than I am a girl.

Me: So, the surgery I had would have been gender-confirming for you?

Jess: And I thought you'd probably have some cool scars. But I have talked to other people who have gone through this, I mean, knowing so many Jewish women. And I know that they're sad.

It was interesting to me how consistent Jess's point of view remained over ten years. Telling her seemed unobjectionable for her back in 2015, and as she reported nothing has changed for her over the past decade. Not only wasn't she disgusted by my surgical history, but she was also jealous. Years before my operations, she had invited me to a game of "I'll show you mine if you show me yours", around the issue of childhood sexual abuse and I had refused to play. I believe that I was likely influenced in disclosing to Jess the story of my mastectomy (without having been fully conscious of it) by lack of conviction that I had made the right decision back in the beginning of the treatment when I would not tell her if I had been molested. I acted like a hockey referee who knows he has blown a call: on a subsequent stoppage of play he may favor the team he had previously ruled against. I suppose that I felt that I could offer her my self-disclosure as a sort of consolation prize.

Patricia

The motivation I felt to tell the one other patient to whom I had disclosed relatively soon after my surgery was different. I began working with Patricia more than 20 years ago when she was pregnant with her second child. She was referred to me for psychopharmacological evaluation, but we started a weekly therapy, then increased to twice-weekly treatment. Some years later, one of her children and one of mine ended up being friendly as they had ended up in overlapping social circles, thus I was worried that Patricia would find out in passing from someone else about my surgery.

I wanted to feel as clear as I could back in 2009 that my choice to disclose wasn't a rationalization, so I didn't tell her immediately when I returned from the month away. I decided to wait and watch her to try to assess her level of wish to know more about what had been going on with me. During an appointment about a year after the surgery, she admitted that because I was "smaller", she had been worrying that I had cancer and was "really sick". I decided I would try to allay her fears with disclosure about the surgery. I told her the facts: I did not have cancer; I had inherited a gene mutation. I had chosen prophylactic mastectomies to try to avoid getting cancer. She seemed relieved. We seldom talked about the surgery or her reaction to it in the years to come.

The treatment had been (and still is) a "supportive therapy". Though of course there have always been currents of transference and countertransference, we have used the interpersonal field less to examine and deepen the treatment and more to nurture and sustain it. She and I still meet twice per week.

Here are excerpts from our recent conversation:

Me: I remember thinking we were in the same community so you might hear it from one of the kids. It's a little hard for me to remember the details and I wouldn't be surprised if you don't, but I guess I'm curious about whether you think that that disclosure negatively impacted you, was neutral, or more net positive? What was your experience of that?

Patricia: I remember asking you if you had reconstructive surgery and you told me, "Yes! And they're awesome!" [We both laugh]. It was a fairly uncommon situation where you know our kids are around the same age and the team and all of that stuff, so you know I was glad to know that. I do remember thinking and you know I'm not scrutinizing people's bodies, but for some reason I just was like oh there's something here and I can't remember how, I mean, how that came about, but I was really affected. It didn't affect me negatively, but it was really, you know, wrenching for me. It was good information to have. I always saw you as a human, but yeah, net positive.

Me: It sounds to me like what you're saying is that the experience of me as a human being: as part of your community, as someone vulnerable, did not destabilize the treatment.

Patricia: Yes, right.

Me: As I remember, I just kind of picked my way through with what felt right. I don't know. It just felt that I was "reading the room" or something like that because I sort of suspected that it would be fine for you– it wouldn't shift the experience of the treatment for you unduly. It wouldn't ruin it for you, which sounds like that feels true to you.

It turns out that Patricia had been worried about my health but didn't feel like she had the right to ask for at least for a year. Ten years after I answered her concerns about my health with self-disclosure, she confirmed that she had felt relieved to know that I didn't have cancer as she had feared.

She also remembered a detail that I had no memory of – my joke about my reconstructed breasts being "awesome!" I suspect that this is how I reassured her that I was really ok–not too sad and vulnerable to function and take care of her. The joke also served as a reminder that we share an appreciation for a certain style of humor.

Linda

At that time of my surgeries, I was a candidate at the psychoanalytic institute and had two patients in psychoanalysis. When I told one of them, a woman in her 50s, that I'd be out of work for a month, she quickly replied: "We don't need to talk about it". By the time I presented the original version of this paper at the National Psychoanalytic Meeting in 2014, five years after the surgery, she had still not asked why I was away. For me, this felt like a straightforward situation. She didn't seem to want to know; I didn't tell her. Her wishes also were a good fit for my formulation of her dynamics. I didn't want her recreating with me the complicated parentification that she had experienced with her mother. But unlike for Jess and Patricia, (as I learned when I told her about the new project) Linda's wishes were a lot more complex than I had understood at the time.

Linda: I think all you told me was that you were having elective surgery.

Me: And you said, "we don't have to talk about that".

Linda: Yeah, but I knew– because well, yeah, let's not talk about it now.

Me: You knew because you heard from somebody? [Linda and my husband had worked for the same institution].

Linda: I have this memory of maybe seeing, I guess I knew what your car was, like seeing your car there, like your husband drove the car to work. I thought–if he's here, then she's okay because he can, you know, be here. I don't know, something like that. Does that make sense? No. I do remember someone asking him how you were doing. I remember hearing– I mean, not totally hearing–bits of what he was talking about. Does that make sense?

Me: That's when I was still out on leave?

Linda: But that's not how I found out. So, in those days, I remember looking at your Facebook page. Oh– you have great privacy–don't worry. All I could see is your cover photo and your profile photo because those are always not non-private, right? But back then I remember looking and it showed some group that you had joined. I mean, I wasn't searching for that, understand. I can't remember exactly what it was– it was that group for people with mutation, like facing your risks–what was it called?

Me: FORCE: Facing Our Risks of Cancer Empowered.

Linda: Right. At the time, I looked it up– like what is that, right?

Me: My girl's wicked *smaht*.

Linda: I know. And then like, you know, soon after that or around I don't remember honestly, I don't remember the timing. How many years ago was that? Like 15, 20 years or something? But whatever, around, you know, at some point after that, then you said, oh, I'm having elective surgery. So, I knew, but you never said anything about it to me.

Me: I don't actually remember telling you.

Linda: It was fairly recently where you just casually mentioned your BRCA mutation. Like you never told me. I just sort of casually acted like I already knew, I don't remember how I reacted. I probably just muttered something like, "I know". Like I think that's probably it. I don't think we got into any detail.

Me: It seems like what I'm hearing is that you liked knowing, but you didn't really want to hear it from me. You liked behind-the-scenes knowing, but you preferred for me not to talk about it with you.

Linda: It was fine knowing, but it wasn't like it gave me like a secret knowledge or something like about you as a human being as opposed to like the person sitting in that chair. And is it good to have that secret knowledge? Was it just interesting? I don't know. It wasn't harmful. I don't think it was harmful. I mean, I don't honestly think about it anymore.

Me: It was a long time ago.

Linda: But I definitely have this memory of overhearing him. Somebody asking like, "how is Michele doing?"

Me: And you had pieced it all together.

Linda: Yeah, I pieced it together. Did you tell all the other children?

It is only because I asked her about her experiences of my self-disclosure for this project that I learned about her sleuthing, but that news didn't surprise me. Linda doesn't easily tolerate being vulnerable. She hates corniness and displays of emotion. Once, I teared up over something she told me, and for years before she'd share anything sad, she'd say, "You're not going to cry, are you?" At the same time, she is curious about me and proud of her online detective skills, so I wasn't surprised that she made it her business to figure out what was going on with me. She remembered that she had "muttered" the words "I know" under her breath, showing her ongoing ambivalence about being seen.

At the end of our conversation, Linda slipped back into one of her ongoing experiences of "sibling rivalry" with my other patients. In a rare moment of vulnerability, she acknowledged her competitive feelings by asking, "Did you tell the other children [my other patients]?" I experienced this moment as a gift, as if she was rewarding my self-disclosure with an intimate admission of her own.

Ilene

I have worked with Ilene, another analytic patient, for more than 20 years. Ilene is a single woman in her 50s, the middle of 13 children. Despite the large number of her siblings, or perhaps because of it, she has always struggled with loneliness.

She has often evinced an intense desire to know details of my private life. A minor example: once in the hallway before her appointment, she overheard the building maintenance man Eddie remark to me: "You scored a deal!" She started the session in despair, burning with curiosity, reluctant to mention it because as she put it, "You'll never tell me anyway . . .". I had been discussing with Eddie a rug I had purchased for my office on Craig's List, a rug Ilene had already had many ideas about. I had no idea whether I would "never tell" her about the rug. No wonder it was so challenging to figure out what to say about an elective surgery that involved my reproductive body parts.

I've felt at times a pressure to participate in a version of a fantasy she shared with me years ago. She wished that she and I could be like a female couple she had seen in a documentary film. The women were lovers and activists during the Nazi regime and were imprisoned together in the same cell for years. Though she was horrified by the idea of the crimes of the Nazi party, and by the idea of prison, she longed to be locked up with me in a mutual love relationship that excluded others.

In early June 2009, I told her about my summer schedule. The following process notes are from an appointment about five weeks before the surgery, about a week after I first told her that I'd be away in July and August. This was the hour in which I told her that my time away was in fact for a medical reason, as she had been suspecting. In retrospect, I think I had been waiting to divine some clear signal from her about what she already knew. Near the beginning of the hour, she had started: "I'm a little worried about you. Maybe I shouldn't be. Maybe you're just living your life . . . I'm trying to be direct and ask you – are you having a medical problem? I don't know – it could be anything . . . you could be having urinary problems, or indigestion . . . It seems like over the past couple of months you've been going to the bathroom more . . .". I responded, perhaps stalling a bit: "You're putting together my going to the bathroom with my being out?" She answered, "I know it doesn't have to be. And again – because I don't know . . . Maybe that seems far-fetched. I felt it would be intrusive for me to say anything about the bathroom – from the tone of your voice, it seems far-fetched". She then said, in a stronger voice, "I think it's time for you to say something". I told her that I was having elective surgery, and that I was hoping to be well and healthy after a period of several weeks of recovery.

In August 2009, she was quite relieved to have me back. She shared her perceptions of my health in a direct manner. Over the years she continued to refer to my surgery, asking whether I might one day "share the information" about what the particular surgery had been with her. She made the argument over the years that by not answering various questions, I contributed to her inability to ascertain reality. She'd press me by saying, "You're trying to teach me how to be in a relationship, but you hold yourself back". Given her desire for information, and her need for a feeling of safety and control, it was hard to feel like I had a clear sense of the meanings and functions of my declining to share details of the surgery, a choice which at times felt calcified.

Sometimes I worried that by not providing the information that she so desperately wanted for years, I was hurting her – pushing her away, sadistically excluding her, and even denying reality in a way that reinforced her obsessional circling. Sometimes it felt like we were playing a sadomasochistic guessing game in which I hid behind my back, just out of reach, the thing she most desired. My occasional experience of dissociation (which felt like projective identification), informed my understanding of her dynamics, and led me to make certain choices about disclosure.

Ilene rarely asks directly for what she wants, but when she does, I can at times feel a kind of pressure, as if she's made an unconscious deal with the world. I imagine that she has a belief that goes something like this: "I ask for so little, so when I do ask for something, you owe it to me". But by not telling Ilene, I've also felt an uncomfortable gratification, a sort of petty pleasure of withholding. With Ilene, I didn't want to feel as if I was being forced. I wanted to resist. I've been perhaps motivated by my wish to sustain a sense of myself as a person with choices. On a more surface level, I've tried to model clear boundaries to try to maintain an unsullied analytic space.

Eventually though, after many years, I did tell Ilene about my surgery. The telling was anticlimactic in the sense that neither of us marked it as a momentous occasion. Then, after several additional years, in the context of this project, I asked her what it had been like for her having had me not disclose for quite some time the details of my surgeries. In the following process notes, we discuss some of the details of my eventually disclosing the information she had wanted to know for so long.

Ilene: I was frustrated that I didn't know what it was, but um you know, because it was such a long time period. It wasn't that you were visibly sick to me, so that was kind of awkward in a way, because you didn't appear to be sick. You didn't seem to be, like, you were in pain or anything. But maybe you were probably going to appointments, but it didn't seem to affect our appointments. You were, you know, going to the appointments–I imagine you had many appointments for that kind of surgery, although I don't know. I remember very well that you said it's not cancer.

Me: Part of it was that I didn't want to foreclose our process. But I also didn't want you to worry unnecessarily.

Ilene: I remember trying to guess what it might be, but I never would have guessed what it ultimately was just because that was not on my mind. I didn't really know anyone that did preventive surgery, even though I knew many people who were Jewish,

Me: What do you remember about how I ended up telling you?

Ilene: Maybe because I bring this up sometimes like I saw you riding on your bike so that I knew you had recovered. You know, you've seen that, because you hadn't been coming to the office on your bike anymore after the surgery. But then, in the Fall I think it was, you had your bike again. And then finally, maybe because I wondered if we were talking about my sister having a mutation, and then me going for genetic testing myself and it could have come up then. I also felt that you were very knowledgeable about oncological things. You are a doctor, but you still seemed like you had the lived experience of being the patient. Like you had real experience.

Me: It's funny after all that–it was such a big deal at the time–and then I finally told you, and now neither of us can really remember the details.

Ilene: You asked me, when you did tell me, was it all right for you to tell me. I said: "well–tell me". I was afraid because it had been withheld for so long. Like–are you really gonna tell me this time? You're not playing with me, are you?

Me: It's interesting that you would think that I would tease you like that.

Ilene: Well, just because of my history, you know. Everyone else always knew, your friends and your family, of course they would know, I mean, I understand that.

Me: So, once you knew, did it feel like a net positive, net negative or pretty neutral?

Ilene: Well, you know, it's kind of like asking me on a scale of one to ten, which I don't like, but I understand why you want to know that . . .

Me: Let me ask a more open-ended question: what was that like?

Ilene: I did like it that you told me because it put things in perspective. It wasn't like this big secret between us. I accepted it that you did not initially tell me. I get that. I came to accept it, but I did like knowing, I do like knowing. It was big. I understood that you went through a big thing. You were very young at that time when that happened. That was very hard. But, it showed me, you're proactive. That was very proactive–the opposite of my own family.

Me: It felt like I modeled something important to you?

Ilene: I mean, you didn't tell me until 15 years later or something. It wasn't like we didn't talk about it.

Me: (laughing) You're saying that 15 years of free association is probably enough?

Ilene was able to tell me that she had experienced my non-disclosure as a painful withholding, a take that did not surprise me. She had spent quite a lot of energy trying to imagine herself into my mind, watching patterns in my behavior such as how I commuted to the office in order to create a theory about my personal experiences. She backfilled the empty space in her understanding of what was going on with me, making her own facsimile of reality.

In our recent conversation about my eventual disclosure, Ilene mostly focused on the experience of having been left out. The details of my health condition mattered less to her than the question of whether I had taken her into my confidence. Like my other patients, in the end she spun her own gold out of the straw of the details I brought to her. In her case, she was impressed by my willingness to be "proactive". She had tried to model her own behavior on my assertive style.

The week after I asked her to revisit the experience of my disclosure, Ilene shared a dream, a new variety of one of her recurrent dreams, showing the ongoing liveliness of the process of disclosure and its sequelae.

Ilene: I had a nice dream last night. You had your long hair back again. We worked at the same place–a very nice hospital, maybe in different departments though. It was a nice feeling.

Me: Camaraderie?

Ilene: Yes. I have to say this: I had some feelings of jealousy because you had other connections.

Me: Yes?

Ilene: But we, just you and I, were chatting in an auditorium. No one was performing, no one was on-stage. Usually in my dreams, you'd be on stage, but we were together in the audience. Equal, but not really because you went off to your other people, but it was still a nice connection. You were still a doctor. [pause]

Me: So, our relationship was mutual, but not parallel?

Ilene: Right. It was good though I guess I felt more myself–I guess that's what self-disclosure is. More yourself. A free exchange. I think your self-disclosure is good for me.

Me: How so?

Ilene: Because I feel freed-up.

Me: The emergence of the new dream may represent the new experience of working together on a project.

Ilene: True!

Me: Perhaps the empty stage represents the future writing project.

Ilene: Right–we're creating something together!

Afterthoughts

It has felt difficult to make a coherent theory of my approach to self-disclosure given that I made different decisions with each of these four patients. Over the years, my decisions about disclosure with these four women have played out on a case-by-case basis. My choices about self-disclosure initially felt unpredictable and verging on random. I self-disclosed to Jess immediately, to Patricia after about a year, to Ilene after many years, and to Linda only in passing, without awareness that I was introducing a novel element to our work together.

Our technique exists under the penumbra of a complex system of influence. The dynamic interaction of our own treatment, our education, and our personalities creates the context for our academic approach. My decisions have been formed within the context of my temperament and character, my understanding of theory, and under the influence of specific moments of my vulnerability and capacity. It is exciting to see that, in retrospect, each of my different approaches made sense within the complex and idiosyncratic system that my patients and I co-created.

Looking at technical choices through the window of self-disclosure has allowed me to notice how the intersubjective field I have established individually with each of my patients led to the emergence of a more coherent and complex system. Within individual relationships with these four patients, and taken as a whole, the work shows radical novelty. New properties appear at higher levels of complexity that were not apparent at lower levels.

At some level, it feels like I blundered through, but I think it's more that with each of these patients as my partners, I *felt* my way through, using intuition as frosting on a cake of preparatory analytic work done over many years. I would name this preparatory work as both positioning myself as a "yes, and" analyst and as trying to model and build a healthy attachment (secure rather than either anxious or avoidant) with my patients. I don't assume that I know better than my patients what is good or right for them. I learned this approach in part from my dyslexic child's teacher at The Carroll School (a school for children with language-based learning differences) during "Parent Visiting Day". We family members had the opportunity to observe our children for a full day of school. I was struck by the supportive and collaborative approach of the teacher responding to the kids as they read. When a child read correctly, the teacher said, "I agree". When the child made a mistake, the teacher responded, "I'm not sure that I agree–what do others think?" I loved this approach. Not only was it not shaming, but it also conveyed a partnership between teacher and students.

Once preparatory work is well underway, improvisation feels less chaotic and risky. In his Substack "Story Club with George Saunders" from May 15, 2025, the author of the novel *Lincoln in the Bardo* explores the question of "Head vs. Heart". He writes:

> *We can't respond to a moment (in a story, or a song, or a movie, or a poem) in the abstract. We have to have a feeling for where we are, for*

> *what hangs in the balance at the moment in the piece . . . Most of my writing, in early drafts, is kind of blurry in this respect . . . Eventually, I'll have a gut feeling of what, say, a certain scene is building toward, and will hone in on it and . . . suddenly that feeling of what you're calling "heart" comes into the room (the room that is that moment in the story). But the room had to be prepared first.*

So too, for me with my four patients. We knew each other well at the time of my self-disclosure. They trusted me and I trusted them. The telling of what I had done with my body came "suddenly", but only after quite a bit of groundwork.

George Saunders (2025) continues:

> *In the kind of moment [we're] talking about, there's a feeling of spontaneity, a true moment of presence – of being aware, at that moment, of what that moment is – what it represents, in . . . the room . . . For [the thing called heart] to happen, both parties need to be in agreement regarding where they are. They are in a state of mutual clarity about that.*
>
> *And that sort of clarity, in my experience, has to be worked at.*

During my training, I had imagined that I would follow the model of the teachers or writers I was learning from. In my classes, I read classic articles by authors who disclosed even taboo sexual and romantic thoughts. From my naive perspective, I believed that once I had a working theory lodged in my brain, my decisions on disclosure would clearly follow. One of my earliest supervisors held a firm line on non-disclosure: he told me that he did not answer any personal questions, even the question of his country of origin (which patients would not infrequently ask him because of his accent). I couldn't imagine working with this level of austerity. I had an uncomfortably different perspective; I wanted to tell. I found that maintaining strict privacy felt uncomfortable rather than protective. I believe I initially held back in order to counteract what felt like dangerous impulsivity. I knew that disclosing *nothing* would not work for me and my patients, but disclosing *everything* would be equally untenable. I've always tried to balance my sense of proper analytic technique with my own voice.

I picture myself negotiating this dilemma as if I was playing the game Labyrinth. The object of the game is to move a marble along a tilted track suspended over a wooden box by using knobs on either side of the box. The maze is interpolated with holes, so that lurching too far one way or another leads to failure. Success takes dexterity and careful timing.

I offer these four vignettes as examples of four different maze patterns. When I revisited my self-disclosure with each of the patients I had presented years earlier, I was gratified to find that each of them felt pleased with how we had negotiated the puzzle. Perhaps this capacity for mutually satisfying work influenced each of their decisions to stay in treatment with me despite the disruption caused first by my leave and then by my self-disclosure.

Note

1 A version of this paper was presented at the 2014 national meetings of the American Psychoanalytic Association.

Reference

Saunders, G. (2025, May 15). Office hours. *Story Club with George Saunders* (blog), *Substack*. georgesaunders.substack.com/p/office-hours-bb8.

Coda

Stephanie R. Brody

Dear Reader:

It is inevitable that dilemmas of self-disclosure will occur in the clinical setting. Unlike almost every human relationship, in psychotherapy and psychoanalysis, the dyad is likely, at some point, to struggle with the structured and defined lopsidedness of the relationship. One shares all, the other listens. One expresses fears, longings, regrets. The other absorbs, learns, wonders. One dreams, mourns, explores. The other responds, echoes, engages. They struggle, question, provoke, create. They travel through history, memory, fantasy and create meaning in the narrative of words, feelings, and of life itself. Over time, each one changes. The lopsidedness becomes more pronounced as the context of external life evolves, as complexity becomes layered, and paths diverge. But still, the connection deepens, the pair know each other, in ways that defy facts and information. The continuity remains, but changes are inescapable. The individual who does not share, cannot help but reveal and be known. The one who has shared, accepts the difference, acknowledges the benefits and lives with mystery. Yet as encounters with unsettling, unexpected, and likely momentous intrusions occur, there are expectations, disappointments, and surprises.

And as this collection of self-disclosure narratives was being finalized, the cosmic sniper sent me a surprise, an opportunity to address the topic, in real time. No hypothetical here – immediate, thoughtful, and personal action was required. Over 20 years have passed since the event that led to the writing of my book, *Entering Night Country*, the discussion group that evolved from that challenge, and *this* book about disclosure. Living out the vulnerability of the analyst, and our humanness in the context of our intimate work, is alive with me now. On the precipice of surgery and facing unsettling ambiguity, I note that any quandaries about disclosure or non-disclosure have disappeared. Then as now, I believe that to be secretive about a personal fact that would impacts a treatment is an analytic evasion, an artifact of theory and practice. Non-disclosure serves to bolster the analyst's wish for omnipotence and protects from the discomforts of frailty. It is a hubris that has been cast as a benefit to the patient. Then, as now, I have

DOI: 10.4324/9781003584803-18

held firmly to the belief that questions can be asked, and will be, though I cannot always give answers for what is not yet known. In each dyad, then as now, the facts and impact were processed within a psychic reality that was meaningful and unique. Though the thread of reality maintained a presence, at times vivid, at times subtle, analytic work was, and is still, possible. The transference remained assuredly, and fascinatingly, hardy, then as now, as I believed it would. Experience has allowed me to carefully consider what entails the affective, factual, symbolic and unconscious disclosures, and how to understand and manage their inevitability. But now, immersed again, I realize how I struggled those decades ago with *my own version of omnipotence* – my fortitude (cracked), my timeline for recovery (too short), my self-sufficiency (an illusion).

After many professional discussions, an ongoing personal analysis, my willingness to accept my fault lines, and ultimately, my impermanence, it has been no less scary, but somewhat easier to bear my new reality and tell the truth. With the scaffolding of my peer groups, who have received my news with thoughtful, loving perspectives, and concrete assistance, I enter now into a new phase of clinical work and professional identity. A new night country. My disclosure is partial, because there is still uncertainty – a reflection of life itself. As I speak to each patient, I feel free to explore the topic of loss, past and current, the possibility of my absence, temporary or permanent, and the turbulence of the era in which we do this intimate work together. Every person, colleagues included, has a singular reaction, and processes the news differently. The hardiness of transference and psychic reality is confirmed, once again. This time, I have committed to enlisting the help of colleagues who will provide coverage and care during my absence. It is a comfort to me, not an exposure. So it is that within this new vulnerability that I have found my competence – to continue my analytic work, to adhere to the analytic identity that represents what I can do and accept what I cannot. To be analytic is also to be human; to face the wish for omnipotence, and its impossibility, in the world of uncertainty. Being human presents us with a tough and wonderful reality – our existence is but a random accident that we may, with enough luck and fortitude, fulfil, with fruitful impact, and relationships that are full of love. But, Readers, it is not for the faint of heart.

This collection of stories are vivid descriptions of deeply challenging clinical encounters. Each reflect the uniqueness of each therapeutic dyad, as well as the endlessly varied meaning of therapist self-disclosure in our profession. They are shared here, with my gratitude: for the generosity, authenticity and integrity of each contributor. I emphasize as well, the individuals who have brought us their pains and struggles and have committed to the transformative process of self-reflection, empathy and personal knowledge that we know is life-altering. We analysts are privileged to be in a profession that is willing to take on the exigencies and narratives of many lives, with individuals who are willing to trust us in this lopsided intimacy. As you enter the narratives, some fraught with pain, frustration, and uncertainty, you will likely have questions and opinions about the facts that have been presented here. It is my sincere hope that, when you collide with such a moment in your life and work, this book will have prepared you to face the facts, neither right nor wrong, but always evocative, and rich with possibility.

Stephanie R. Brody ~ January 23, 2026

Index

For Product Safety Concerns and Information please contact our EU representative GPSR@taylorandfrancis.com
Taylor & Francis Verlag GmbH, Kaufingerstraße 24, 80331 München, Germany

www.ingramcontent.com/pod-product-compliance
Lightning Source LLC
LaVergne TN
LVHW020724290926
849104LV00028B/327
9781032951034